BREAST SELF-EXAMINATION

BREAST SELF-EXAMINATION

ALBERT R. MILAN, M.D.
ILLUSTRATIONS BY THE AUTHOR

LIBERTY PUBLISHING COMPANY

WORKMAN PUBLISHING
NEW YORK

**Library of Congress Cataloging in
Publication Data**
Milan, Albert R
Breast self-examination.

1. Breast—Examination.   2. Self-examination,
Medical.   3. Breast—Cancer—Diagnosis. I.
Title.
[DNIM: 1. Breast neoplasms—Prevention and
control—
Popular works.   WP870 M637b]
RG493.M54   1980   616.99'4490754   79-
56529
ISBN 0-89480-075-2
ISBN 0-89480-124-4 (pbk.)

Cover design: Paul Hanson
Book design: Charles Kreloff

Published in cooperation with
Liberty Publishing Company

Workman Publishing Company
1 West 39 Street
New York, N.Y. 10018

Manufactured in the United States of America

10 9 8 7 6 5 4 3 2 1

ACKNOWLEDGMENTS

This book is dedicated to my many teachers and colleagues who have produced physicians and nurses of impeccable qualifications and who have instilled in their hearts an inspirational quality that life's greatest achievement is to better the quality of life for one's fellow man. A debt of gratitude is owed to my esteemed colleagues, Dr. Edward F. Lewison and Dr. Clifford R. Wheeless, Jr., for their inspiration, encouragement and suggestions in effectively assembling this material; and to Dr. Lawrence E. Holder for his suggestions and review of technical information pertaining to the radiological aspects of material contained in this volume. To the thousands of patients I have had the opportunity to grow up and "mature" with, with whom I have been able to share affectionate laughter as well as heartfelt tears. To those who have helped me, advised me and encouraged me to tell the story like it is, so that their experiences, both joyous and disconsolate, might in some way lighten the burdens of others. To those who are nearest and dearest to me who have proven beyond any shadow of a doubt that cancer is curable, if we are given half a fighting chance to do it. To my life-long secretaries, Mrs. Kathleen Sampson, Mrs. Phyllis Reid, Miss Patty Milan and Mrs. Bobbie Smith, and most importantly to my very dear and devoted wife and daughters whose profound devotion, unselfishness, sacrifices and encouragement have allowed me to assemble this information, hopefully for the betterment of the human race, this book is affectionately dedicated.

A.R.M.

FOR
MARJORIE HALLERAN MILAN

INTRODUCTORY
COMMENTS

Edward F. Lewison, M.D.

Chief, Breast Clinic
Johns Hopkins Hospital

Associate Professor of Surgery
Johns Hopkins University School of Medicine

Clifford R. Wheeless, Jr., M.D.

Chief, Gynecology and Obstetrics
The Union Memorial Hospital

Assistant Professor Gynecology and Obstetrics
Johns Hopkins University School of Medicine

Almost 90,000 American women develop breast cancer every year. Medical experience indicates that 90 percent of these breast cancers are discovered by women themselves—but unfortunately not always in time.

By means of the simple health habit of breast self-examination which is so vividly described in this vital manual, women could discover these lumps in their breasts at the earliest possible time. Mammography is, of course, a most helpful diagnostic aid.

Dr. Albert R. Milan has written and personally illustrated a life-saving little book on breast self-examination. He has made the technique easy to learn and simple to practice.

This well-illustrated book encourages and teaches women to examine their own breasts once a month, just after the menstrual period, and equally important, at regular monthly intervals after the menopause. If a lump is discovered, they should see their doctor without delay.

The author of this book has performed a service to humanity. My sincere congratulations to Dr. Milan for his special interest, dedication and effort in the preparation of this public educational guide. By practicing breast self-examination, women will discover today what would be all too ominous tomorrow.

Edward F. Lewison, M.D.

Successful management of breast cancer requires the mobilization of the combined resources of many disciplines, including the media, the cancer societies, the medical profession and, most importantly, the public. Detection of this disease in its advanced stages requires no special skill. The chances of cure are directly dependent upon how early the disease is detected and treated. The theme of this book is directed at early detection.

Since it is logistically impossible for the physician to seek out the patients with the early clues, it becomes the responsibility of the patient to perform this detective work upon herself. Though the procedure is not difficult to master, a graphic and comprehensible text which the woman can study in the privacy of her home appears to be a very valid first step. Dr. Milan has succeeded in writing and illustrating this much needed manual for the layman, covering the procedure in a simple step-by-step manner. Not only has he attempted to clarify the significance of some of the early clues, but also to emphasize the importance of utilizing the expertise of the physician in the critical decision-making process.

Of those breast lumps discovered by doctors, over 90 percent are detected by the obstetrician-gynecologist. Thus the onus not only of detecting this condition early, but also of making the proper primary decision weighs heavily upon his diagnostic acumen and skill. It is his responsibility to mobilize, synthesize and utilize every available facet of modern medical technology in the early detection of this disease. The author has distilled out the most important features encountered in a lifetime of experience to facilitate the teaching of the early detection of breast cancer by self-examination to every woman who will take the time to learn.

This small volume fills a critically needed void which hopefully will be the educational vehicle needed to spare the unnecessary loss of many thousands of lives to an awesome enemy.

Clifford R. Wheeless, Jr., M.D.

CONTENTS

AUTHOR'S PREFACE

If a magic genie could grant us two very simple wishes, we would be able to save the lives of as many as 40,000 American women every year. The first wish is that all breast cancers would be detected in their earliest stages. The second is that treatment would be sought at the earliest possible moment after a potential problem is detected. One might casually evaluate these wishes as insignificant; in reality, they are of monumental importance. Despite great efforts and the investment of tremendous funds and countless man-hours, our death rate from breast cancer is essentially the same today as it was in 1930. Ironically, both these wishes could be easily realized if only we could convince people that breast cancer, when detected and treated early, is curable.

This work is an illustrated presentation of a Breast Self-Examination Procedure that is reliable, easily performed and without cost. A lifetime in the clinical practice of diagnostic gynecology and obstetrics has served as the basis on which to assemble the best available methods of searching out the subtle clues essential for the meticulous detection of our elusive enemy in its most curable stages. The author has been singularly blessed by the opportunity to study under two of the great founding fathers of the philosophy of breast self-examination, Dr. Hugh Auchincloss and Dr. Cushman Haagenson, both of Columbia University. These fine gentlemen have devoted their lives to improving the lot of the victims of breast cancer. Dr. Haagenson's textbook on the subject remains the reference bible for all who have any dealings with this disease. In his own inimitable way, Dr. Auchincloss was able to kindle a spark of hope in the hearts of many young medical students whose outlook toward the cure of cancer was skeptical at best.

A sincere endeavor has been made to describe and explain many of the harmless findings in an effort to reduce panic. Wherever possible, I have illustrated logical explanations for these clues. Diagrams and descriptions are given so that the reader will know exactly how to proceed and will be able to do so with the utmost confidence. The illustrations are all original, and clearly and succinctly depict certain basic facts. Each has been designed to convey its own message. All have been denuded of cumbersome and irrelevant details. I urge that the entire book be read before the breast self-examination procedure is begun.

It is my profound hope that this work will serve as a reference book for the many women who hunger for guidance in proper examination techniques and interpretation of the more common findings. It is paramount that breast self-examination be learned and practiced at an early age, so that each and every young woman not only will acquire an exceedingly important health habit but also will learn the individualized aspects of her anatomy and its functions. It is only in this manner that she will be able to detect the early and sophisticated changes that might become a threat to her. I pray that nothing worrisome will ever be found. I am confident that if this procedure is performed correctly, the chances of missing anything significant will be exceedingly small. Most important, the more skillful a woman becomes in performing the examination, the more peace of mind she will have in knowing exactly what is there. If the many years that have been spent in the preparation of this work will help to save just one life from this miserable affliction, then I will feel justly rewarded.

BREAST SELF-EXAMINATION

CHAPTER 1
THE IMPORTANCE OF BREAST SELF-EXAMINATION

The war on cancer is a crusade waged by all of mankind against a universal enemy. A vast body of knowledge, representing the combined efforts of every nation on this planet, has been assembled in an attempt to fit together the bizarre and complex pieces of the cancer puzzle. Yet for those who have spent their lives wrestling with the problems of this disease, the dream of a cure must be tempered by some sobering thoughts. Assume that we had in our possession today an absolute, positive method of arresting every conceivable type of cancer. Important and unanswered questions would still haunt us. How would we know whom to cure? How would we know who has what kind of cancer and in what stage? Thus, even when the exact knowledge of how to cure cancer is at our disposal, we will have to revert back to basics and confront the problems of early detection. The greatest single thread of truth about the cancer enigma is that many cancers are curable if the disease is detected early and if it is treated aggressively without delay. Only then will we be able to stave off the irreversible organ devastation that is the hallmark of the disease.

The importance of early detection is painfully apparent in the case of breast cancer. Despite the brilliant advances in medical knowledge and skills, the mortality rate from breast cancer has changed very little during the past half-century. One hundred and eight thousand new cases of breast cancer are discovered each year, and of those women involved, 40 to 50 percent will be alive after five years. For those individuals in whom the tumor is small (marble-size or smaller) and there is no evidence of spread, the chances of survival approach 80 to 90 percent.

The difference between these percentages represents about 40,000 lives per year—the difference between what we are actually doing and what we could be doing to arrest the cancer if it were detected in its earliest stages.

We have the capabilities and the technology to drastically change this situation. First and foremost, however, the efforts of the medical profession and of the general public must be combined to overcome certain basic attitudes toward cancer, namely, fear and its compatriot, procrastination. In fact, one cannot afford to be afraid. The cruel realities of life teach us that breast cancer is among the greatest killers of women. One out of fifteen women will eventually be victimized by this awesome disease.

Failure to detect breast cancer in its earliest stages is the greatest single redeemable sin in the entire cancer confrontation. Another atonable sin in the present-day approach to this tragedy is our failure to accept the fact that a problem exists once a suspicious change has been discovered. These are two very basic reasons for the mediocre results being achieved in the battle against cancer. It is a sad commentary that the average interval between the moment a suspicious sign is discovered and the first visit to a physician is five to six months.

This period of procrastination may allow the early localized disease enough time to convert into one that has spread. When the localized condition is treated, the chances of survival are excellent. Wiping out the tremendous loss of life caused by fear is a lofty goal indeed, but it is attainable. Mustering the combined forces of a well-informed general public and an aggressive medical profession is a mandatory first step.

Once the barrier of fear has been conquered, the question becomes "How can we best protect ourselves?" One of the highest priorities of cancer researchers is the development of a simple, accurate, inexpensive and harmless procedure to facilitate the early detection of breast cancer. In the absence of such a test, our survival must depend on the use of existing procedures. Ranking most effective on the list is the simple procedure of breast self-examination. Though it is never too late to introduce this very essential health habit into one's important "musts" for self-preservation, it is best to begin this procedure in early womanhood. It should become as much of an established ritual as is the annual Pap smear and the gynecological examination. One of the gems in the crown of this past century's medical achievements has been the drastic and dramatic decline in the death rate from cervical cancer that has been made possible by the perfection of the Pap smear, regular gynecological examinations and mass screening. The disease is still very much with us and still threatens us; however, when detected in the "brush fire" stage, the devastation and tragedies of the "forest fire" potential can be avoided.

The likelihood of a breast lump being malignant in a woman in her late teens and early twenties is small, but it is possible—and it has happened—though the incidence rises sharply at age thirty-five. Fibroadenomas and fluid-filled cysts are the most common causes for breast lumps in the young woman. For the most part harmless, these "lumps" can, however, attain a substantial size and produce sufficient pressure to destroy much of the normal surrounding breast tissue. When the lump is removed, the breast may be deformed and drastically reduced in size because of the tissue destruction. While the physician may be able to diagnose some of these lumps without surgery, many of them are almost impossible to differentiate accurately by any means other than surgical biopsy.

Much research work has been done on the rate of cell growth. The time required for a tumor to double its volume is known as the ''doubling time.'' Certain very aggressive tumors can double very rapidly; others are very slow. Mathematical calculations based on these doubling times indicate that many breast cancers may have been present for two to eight years before they were large enough to be seen, felt, or detected by mammography. Herein lies one of the critical values of breast self-examination. If a lump is large enough to be detected in a thirty-two-year-old woman, how much time has passed since its inception? Can it be pinpointed at the mid-twenties? It is apparent, then, that the younger the woman is when she begins self-examination, the better. The more familiar she is with every little nodule and peculiarity in her breasts, the more readily will she be able to discover a new and *different* dominant mass or visual change.

If we will ever be able to win this war, we need all the help we can muster from any and every source. A surprising number of women report that the lump in their breast was ''first found by my husband.'' Likewise, husbands may call to make appointments for their wives to check out a worrisome finding. If the woman is too ''spooky'' about doing her own examination, I have recommended that it be done by the husband. Indeed, the men must play a role in this crusade by encouraging their wives to do self-examinations and to have their annual physical exams, by supporting and assisting their wives in this habit in any way humanly possible and by encouraging their mothers and daughters and sisters to do the same. *Everyone* should participate. Above all, we must teach the young to develop this habit at a tender age and to practice it faithfully throughout their lifetime.

Although pain serves as a warning in conjunction with other diseases, unfortunately, with breast cancer, there are no early symptoms to alert us that there might be a problem. Moreover, though many women feel that an annual visit to their physician is sufficient, we have been forced to recognize the fact that lumps can become apparent a few short months after their physician performed an extensive and thorough examination. A diligent and thorough breast self-examination program is therefore the best possible insurance against invasive breast cancer. It costs nothing, it is not time-consuming and it is reliable. And it can spare more lives in one single year than we lost in all the years of the war in Vietnam.

CHAPTER 2
THE TOUCH PICTURE OF THE BREAST

T he reason most often given by new patients for failing to perform breast self-examination is fear: "I'm afraid because I don't know how to do it correctly" . . . "afraid I might find something" . . . "afraid because I won't be able to differentiate what I should and should not be concerned about." Even those women exposed to movies, slide presentations and leaflets on breast self-examination will proceed with the exam using only the bits and pieces they are able to remember. And when they discover something that they are unable to recognize or consider normal, sheer panic will prevail.

It is therefore essential that women have a fundamental understanding of the function of the normal breast and its anatomical structures. Then, armed with these basics, they will be able to fend off many of their unnecessary apprehensions. Naturally, one cannot expect to categorize everything with mathematical correctness. The ideal goal of patient education will have been achieved if a woman is able to discern that which has always been present from that which represents a recent occurrence or change.

It must be remembered that this book is in no way

intended to be a substitute for a visit to the doctor. On the contrary, it supports the commandment that whenever something unusual is found, one must consult her physician at the earliest possible moment. The book is designed as a reference to fill the void experienced by the average woman when she goes home to perform her breast self-examination and cannot recall the details of the movie, the slide presentation or her physician's lecture.

FUNCTION OF THE BREAST

From the earliest stages in the development of the human embryo, certain cells are destined to become the integumentary, or skin structures, which cover the surface of the body. These cells will be further subdivided to develop into specialized structures, such as hair, hair follicles, sweat and oil glands and surface skin. The breasts evolve from some of the sweat and oil gland cells and ultimately become highly specialized organs, the primary function of which is to nurture the offspring. Just as many substances consumed by human beings are secreted into the sweat glands, so it is that some of them can also find their way into the breast secretions. A plausible theory on the development of breast cancer is that some carcinogenic chemicals may find their way into these breast secretions, remain there for long periods of time and affect certain surrounding cells by converting them into cancer cells.

Through the eons of human evolution, the breasts have become much more than basic structures for nurturing the young. They are intimately integrated with the rest of the body so that we can expect responses from complex changes in the biochemical, hormonal, neurological, emotional and reproductive systems. Additionally, the breasts have played a significant role in the courtship between man and woman, and have been displayed and flaunted in various fashions to attract the eye of a potential mate. Likewise, the breasts assume an important function in attaining sexual satisfaction. Despite arguments to the contrary, our modern society has oriented the major functional role of the female breasts to that of aesthetic sex objects.

ANATOMICAL FACTORS

Normal breasts are composed of milk glands, fat lobules, fibrous tissue bands, blood vessels and skin. The milk gland portion of the breast is similar to a bunch of grapes (see Fig. 1). Many tiny grapelets are bunched together in small clusters, each of which is composed of multiple gland cells whose function is to produce the breast milk. A collecting system empties the contents of each cluster of cells into a small stemlike duct. This duct leads to a larger duct, and that to a still larger one, until the contents ultimately drain into the nipple. There may be ten to twenty large terminal ducts that discharge from the nipple.

The only muscles in the breasts are the tiny erectile muscles within the nipples. The breasts are situated on the surface of the large pectoral muscles. These are the heavy-work muscles located on the front of the chest that control the upper arm and shoulder. Movement of these muscles causes the overlying breasts to move with them. The attachment of each breast to the muscle beneath is usually quite loose and the entire breast moves with it as a unit. Certain conditions, such as scar tissue or tumor growths, may cause the breast to adhere to this muscle in isolated areas. As the muscle attached to this spotty area is moved, the breast will change shape or a dimple will occur.

The architectural form of the breast is maintained by interwoven semi-elastic fibrous partitions and bands that were first described in 1845 by Sir Astley Cooper and bear

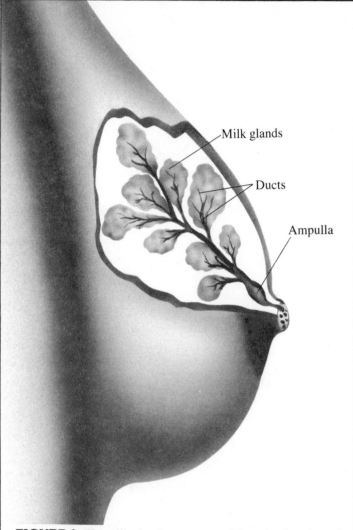

Milk glands

Ducts

Ampulla

FIGURE 1. The milk glands are comparable to tiny bunches of grapes interconnected by small stemlike ducts. The smaller ducts lead to progressively larger ones, which ultimately empty into the nipple. The terminal ducts are situated beneath the areola and form a bulbous swelling known as the ampulla. The prominent ampullas can be felt as slippery pea-sized swellings, arranged in a circular pattern in the outer rim of the areola.

the name "Cooper's ligaments." The breast is constructed like a sponge, honeycombed with large intercommunicating pockets that contain the milk glands and fat lobules. The milk ducts pass through these interconnecting pockets as they convey the breast milk to the nipple (see Fig. 2). If all the milk glands and surrounding fat were removed from these pockets, only the thin, lacelike Cooper's ligaments would remain and the structural framework would then flatten out like a deflated balloon.

The significance of this framework has not been utilized to its fullest extent in the establishment of techniques for the early detection of breast cancer. The presence of a tumor mass within the spongelike framework of the breast causes an entanglement of the fibers of the Cooper's ligaments (see Fig. 3). As a result, not only is there a loss of the elastic qualities of these fibers, but physical distortion of the shape of the breast is likely to occur. The fibers in the affected area become fixed either to the skin or to the pectoral muscle, while the remainder of the breast is still soft, pliable and freely movable. Thus, if we alter the position of the movable portions of the breast by various maneuvers, we can focus on a new dimple, indentation, retraction (pulling) or distortion that is capable of supplying us with important early clues to a possible cancer.

On the other hand, the elastic partitions can be adversely distorted by a host of benign conditions that most certainly should be ruled out before any conclusions are reached. A few of the more common causes are: residual scar tissue from previous breast surgery, breast abscesses, mastitis, previous injuries, and the injection of various augmentation materials into the breasts.

It is important to emphasize again that we must concentrate on a recent *change* rather than on the presence of any preexistent normal variants. The changes become very significant if they were not present in the past and if there is no good explanation for their presence now.

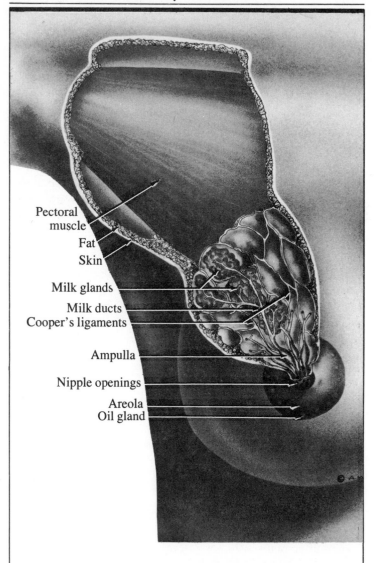

Pectoral muscle
Fat
Skin
Milk glands
Milk ducts
Cooper's ligaments
Ampulla
Nipple openings
Areola
Oil gland

FIGURE 2. The breast is composed of compartments formed by the lacelike fibrous partitions known as ''Cooper's ligaments.'' These partitions give the breast its rounded form. Each compartment is filled with milk glands and fatty tissue.

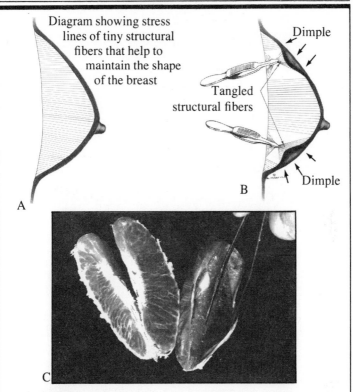

FIGURE 3. Diagram A is an oversimplification of the elastic fibrous partitions (Cooper's ligaments) that make up the intrinsic architectural structure of the breasts. One end of these fibrous partitions is attached to the under surface of the skin, while the other is connected to the surface of the chest wall.

In diagram B, stress is applied to various groups of these fibrous bands with imaginary tweezers to demonstrate the mechanics of how dimples, indentations and distortions can occur by pulling or entangling these bands.

An analogy drawn from nature (diagram C) shows two sections of an orange with the partition membrane of one of the sections dissected from the orange pulp. If the pulp is carefully removed from within this membranous sac, the structure will collapse. The milk glands and fatty tissues within the pockets formed by the Cooper's ligaments are comparable to the fleshy part of the orange. The function of the fatty tissue appears to be one of "upholstering," or padding.

THE TOUCH PICTURE OF BREAST TISSUE

An understanding of the anatomical structures of the breast makes it a bit easier to comprehend the touch picture of the normal breast. It is difficult even for a trained examiner to differentiate between milk glands, milk ducts and fat lobules. All these structures are soft, they all impart a granular and slippery sensation and they are usually movable. A simple experiment can be an aid in learning approximately what the average breast should feel like. First, fill a plastic food bag with a warm gelatin solution. Add some partially cooked rice kernels. After this mixture has cooled and firmed up, feel the contents of the bag through its outer surface. It will have a granular texture comparable to that of an average breast. Toward the end of the normal menstrual cycle and just before the flow is to start, the kernel-sized breast granules enlarge so they may approach the size of small peas.

Many women commonly have a benign condition known as cystic mastitis, which is characterized by the presence of a multitude of different-sized tender breast cysts. In these individuals, the pea-sized granules may increase to the size of peanuts and occasionally larger. The swollen milk glands are usually quite tender and are responsible for the generalized soreness of the breasts experienced in the premenstrual phase of the cycle. This response is not abnormal; it is produced by the normal body hormones associated with ovulation. One can readily see from this explanation why breast examination in the later part of the cycle is not advisable. It is uncomfortable and can produce unwarranted anxiety because of the presence of the many enlarged and engorged tender milk glands and ducts. For these reasons, the best time to examine the breasts is in their resting phase, during the first week after the menstrual flow has subsided.

The normal milk glands, fat lobules and enlarged

ducts are usually smooth and slippery. Conversely, many of the hard, fixed and immovable lumps in the breast may not be harmless and therefore require further investigation. Most malignant lumps are fixed; however, many fixed lumps are harmless. It is very difficult to be certain on the basis of tactile sensation alone. There is only one way of being certain and that is by adequate biopsy. An estimated 60 to 80 percent of all breast lumps removed as surgical biopsies are found to be harmless.

A simple method of distinguishing the tactile sensation imparted by the harmless slippery breast cysts and ducts from that of the firm, fixed (and possibly harmful) lumps is the "eye and nose" test. Close one eye and place your fingertip on the eyelid. Gently move the eyelid over the surface of the eyeball (see Fig. 4A). You will sense that the eyeball is slippery and movable, and that the lid glides smoothly over it. Next, pinch the eyelid to lift it away from the surface of the eyeball. It lifts freely and easily. These are the sensations imparted by the normal milk glands and ducts of the breast, as well as by many of the harmless breast cysts.

Now place the ball of your fingertip on the end of your nose (see Fig. 4B). Try to move the nasal skin beneath your finger without moving the tip of your nose. It won't go. It is fixed and the tip of the nose moves with the skin. Try to lift the skin on the tip of your nose by pinching it between your fingertips, as you did with your eyelid. It cannot be lifted. This is a very important differentiating feature.

Normal milk glands, milk ducts and cysts are unattached like the eye (see Fig. 5A). Any lump in your breast that does not move, that is attached to the skin and above which you are unable to pinch the skin (see Fig. 5B) should be examined by your physician without delay. It should also be noted again that while most of the smooth, slippery lumps are harmless, a small number of them are not. The decision making should be left to the expertise of your physician.

EYELID AND NOSETIP TEST

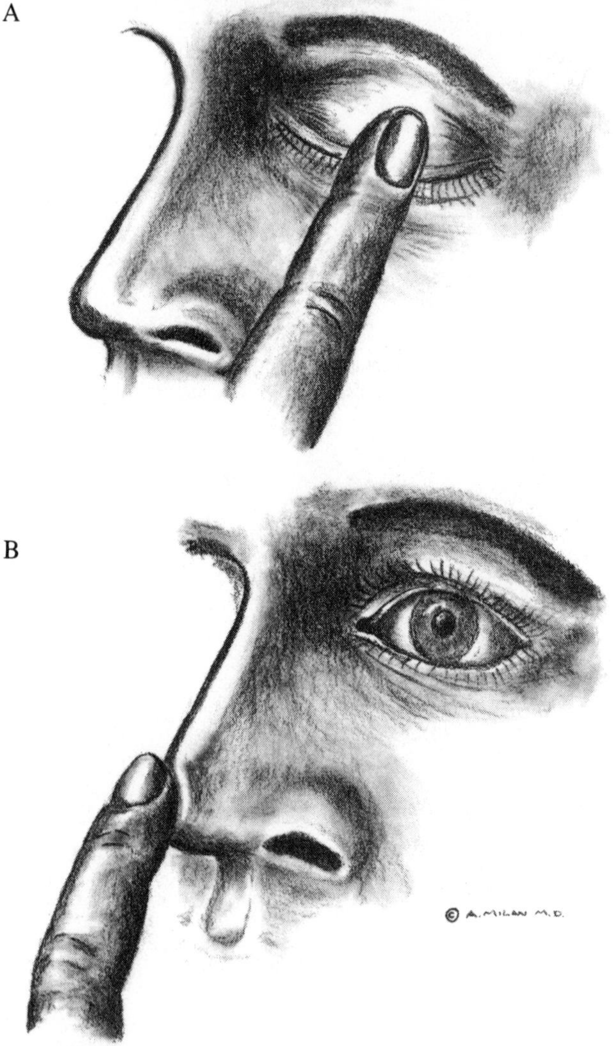

A

B

© A. MILAN M.D.

FIGURE 4. Place the flat of the fingertip on the eyelid (A). Roll the lid over the smooth slippery eyeball. Now try to move the skin of the tip of the nose over the underlying cartilage in a similar manner (B). The cartilage is adherent and moves only with the skin.

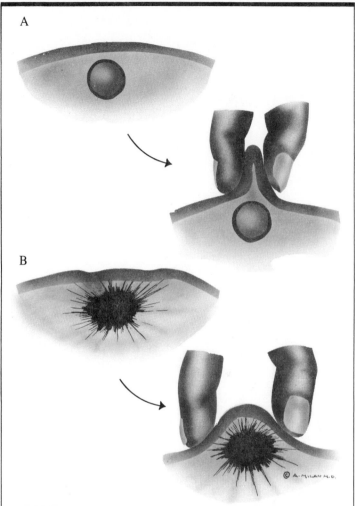

FIGURE 5. A slippery, movable lump under the skin is compared with a lump that is fixed. The slippery lump (A) seems to lie free under the surface of the skin. The skin is easily rolled over it and is readily lifted away from the lump by pinching, just as the eyelid can be lifted over the eyeball. The fixed lump (B) seems to be attached by bands or fibrous tentacles. When the skin is pinched, it resists the pull away from the lump. A fixed lump is an important indication for an immediate visit to your physician.

CHAPTER 3
BREAST SELF-EXAMINATION: PALPATION

E ach and every woman should make it a health ritual to examine her breasts once a month. There are no magic formulas and no special abilities or instruments needed to effectively perform the exam. One depends primarily on two God-given faculties: the sense of touch and the visual sense. A large mirror and about ten minutes of time per month are the basic requirements.

The best time for the younger, premenopausal woman to perform the exam is during the week immediately after the menstrual flow has stopped. Postmenopausal and post-hysterectomy women should perform the exam on the first calendar day of each month. In the case of post-hysterectomy patients whose ovaries have not been removed, cyclic changes are likely to occur and a time should be selected during the month when the individual is devoid of ''premenstrual'' symptoms and particularly tender swollen breasts.

The monthly breast self-examination is best carried out in the morning. The first part of the examination is done while in the shower, the second part while lying flat in bed, and the third while standing erect before a large mirror. Details of each of these procedures will be described in this chapter and the next. It is most important to establish a definite technique and then adhere strictly to it.

There may be a feeling of uncertainty after the first self-examination; however, each time it is done, confidence develops until finally the fundamentals are mastered and a sense of well-being takes over. Confidence comes with practice and with familiarity with one's body.

LEARNING "HOW TO FEEL"

Certain basic principles must be learned before undertaking breast self-examination. These are not difficult to master; rather, they are readily acquired after a bit of practice. What we are trying to feel is usually not sitting on the surface of the skin. Instead, it is below the surface and, sometimes, very deep indeed.

Nerve endings designed to function in the sensory capacity of touch, or the tactile sensation, are found on the entire surface of the body. Large numbers of these nerve endings are present in the pads of the fingertips. They are part of a complex and sophisticated hookup with the brain that is capable of immediately delivering a computerized picture of the physical properties of anything they come in contact with. The medical term for examining something by utilizing the sense of touch is *palpation*. Assuming there are a limited number of these touch receptors present in our fingertips, we must avoid dissipating them by simultaneously asking them to do many things. Rather, we want to concentrate on the physical properties of anything and everything below the surface of the skin. If we let the fingertips slide over the skin, we can tell if it is rough or smooth, dry or oily, hot or cold, hairy or slippery, and if there are warts, moles or scales on the skin surface. We can learn little or nothing, however, about lumps, thickenings or granules below the surface. By contrast, if we immobilize the skin with the fingertips and move it over the underlying structures, we avoid wastage of any of the

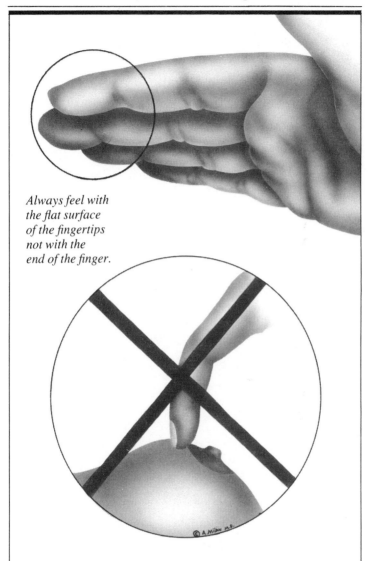

*Always feel with
the flat surface
of the fingertips
not with the
end of the finger.*

FIGURE 6. The most sensitive tactile areas are located in the "palmar pads" of the fingertips. When performing breast self-examination, always use two or three fingers utilizing the flat surfaces of the fingertips. Avoid using the end of the finger. A long fingernail interferes with the sense of touch.

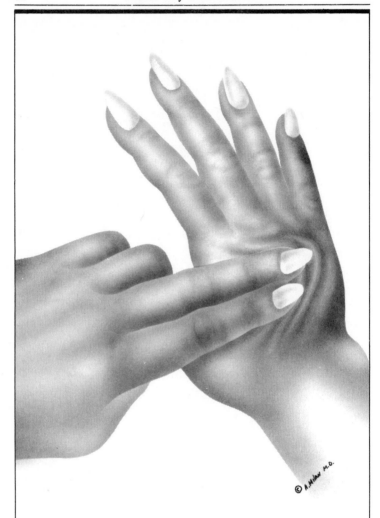

FIGURE 7. Allowing the two examining fingers to glide over the surface of the skin will give you information about the texture of the surface of the skin but only a crude impression about what is beneath the surface.

Press down gently with the fingertips so that the skin moves with the fingers. Roll the skin around in small circular patterns over the underlying bones, joints and tendons. Imagine that the skin is not there and that you have eyes in your fingertips.

tactile nerve pathways on the surface properties and allow all of them to be concentrated on feeling what is situated in the breast below the surface of the skin.

One of the most frequent errors made in performing breast self-examination is digging into the breast tissues with the *end* of the fingertip or fingernail. The most sensitive areas of touch are situated in the "palmar pads" of the fingers (see Fig. 6). It is wiser to use two or more fingers together instead of a single finger. If an irregularity is felt, it can be bobbled between the fingertips to yield information about size, shape, mobility, firmness and other factors.

A simple method of practicing the palpation technique is to place two fingers of one hand on the back surface of the other. Gently and without moving the skin, allow the pads of these two fingers to slide lightly back and forth over the surface of the hand. At the same time, try to feel some of the prominences of the tendons and bones beneath the surface. Now, instead of allowing the fingertips to slide *over* the surface, gently press them downward so that the skin is immobilized and is moved with the fingertips over the underlying structures (see Fig. 7). Rotating the fingers in small circular patterns, advance from one area to the next until you have covered the back of the entire hand. You will quickly become aware of how much more can be learned about what is below the surface when you move the skin with your "feeling" fingers.

The same technique is used in examining the breasts (see Figs. 8A and 8B). Fix the skin with the flat of two or more fingers and use small rotary movements.

It is important to remember that minor changes take place within the breast structure on a daily basis, particularly in the premenopausal woman. Harmless cysts occur commonly in the later days of the menstrual cycle and usually will disappear when the menstrual flow is completed. If they persist, they should be investigated. (Details will be given later on how to differentiate these cysts from

CORRECT

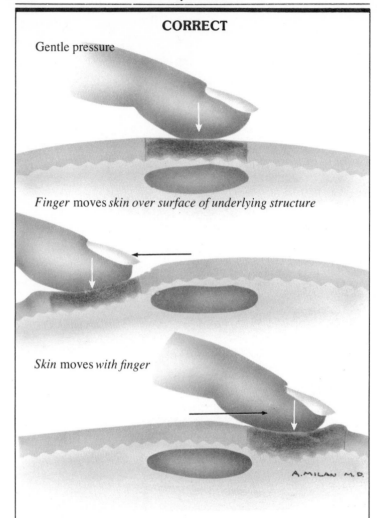

Gentle pressure

Finger moves *skin over surface of underlying structure*

Skin moves *with finger*

A. MILAN M.D.

FIGURE 8A. If the fingertip is allowed to slide over the surface of the skin, little or no information can be acquired about the structures below the surface. One can learn all about the texture of the surface of the skin, but this is not of primary importance. The tactile nerve endings of the fingertips are "preoccupied with surface sensations" and are less likely to pick up the deeper sensations with which we are concerned in breast self-examination.

INCORRECT

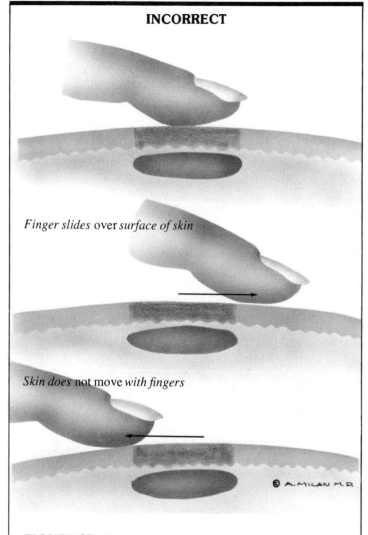

Finger slides over *surface of skin*

Skin does not move *with fingers*

FIGURE 8B. On the other hand, when gentle pressure is applied with the examining finger on the shaded area of skin, this area is moved back and forth over the underlying lump. The lump is examined carefully until it can be defined for size, shape, softness or hardness, surface characteristics and movability. Always feel with the flat surface of the fingertip and preferably with two or more fingers.

more significant findings.) The differential diagnosis of what is taken to be a simple breast cyst is not always easy and may require other investigative procedures. The physician may draw upon any number of diagnostic procedures in his decision making.

EXAMINATION IN THE SHOWER

The first part of breast self-examination is performed in the shower in the upright position. Thoroughly covering the breasts with soap facilitates the examination. Each breast is examined by the opposite hand; i.e., the left breast is examined with the right hand and vice versa. The arm on the side being examined should be raised and placed comfortably on the head or on the back of the neck. For the individual with pendulous breasts, a one-handed examination may reveal very little. In this situation, it is best to immobilize the breast by lifting it with the palm of the hand on the side being examined as if it were placed upon a shelf (see Fig. 9). With the other hand, feel the top surface of the breast with the top hand, then hold the top hand steady and feel for any lumps with the bottom hand. Repeat the procedure on the opposite side. Similarly, the pendulous breast may be backed against the chest wall while it is examined with the other hand (see Fig. 10).

THE CIRCULAR PATTERN METHOD

It is essential that the entire breast be examined and that nothing be missed. Use a systematic pattern that covers the entire chest area, from the collarbone to just below the breast line, from the armpit around to the midline (see Fig. 11). Of the many methods proposed to help guarantee this very essential requirement, the concentric circle method developed and promoted by the American Cancer Society

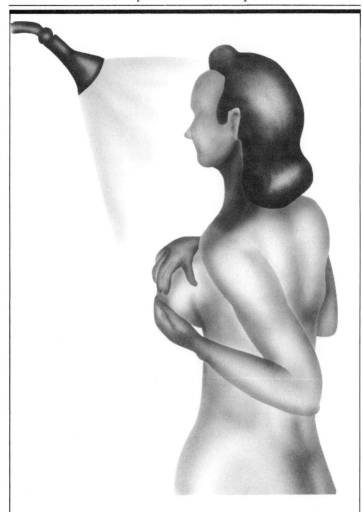

FIGURE 9. Covering the breasts with a generous soapy lather seems to enhance one's tactile sense. If the breasts are small, a one-handed examination will suffice. The arm on the side being examined is raised above the head, while the breast is examined with the opposite hand. If the breasts are large, it is better to use both hands. One hand is used to support the breast, while the other hand examines. Examine by having the breast immobilized either between the two hands or between one hand and the chest wall.

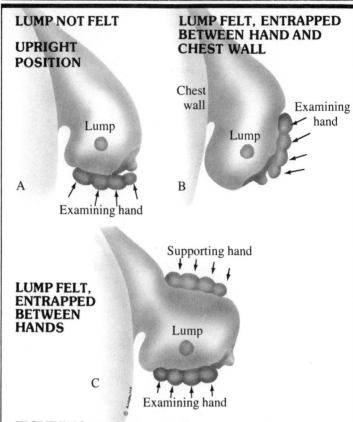

LUMP NOT FELT

UPRIGHT POSITION

LUMP FELT, ENTRAPPED BETWEEN HAND AND CHEST WALL

Lump

Examining hand

A

Examining hand

Chest wall

Lump

Examining hand

B

LUMP FELT, ENTRAPPED BETWEEN HANDS

Supporting hand

Lump

C

Examining hand

FIGURE 10. These diagrams illustrate some of the problems encountered when examining the pendulous breasts while in the upright posture. A small lump is situated just behind the nipple. If only one hand is used and is placed on the under surface of the breast so that it lifts it upward (A), the small lump floats out of the way and is sure to be missed. If, however, the examining hand presses the breast backward, the lump is entrapped between the hand and the chest wall (B), and the chances of detecting it are good. Better still, use one hand as a backstop and the other to do the examining (C). Hold the supporting hand steady and gently roll the fingers of the examining hand in small circular movements until the entire breast area is covered. Then hold the bottom hand steady as the supporting hand and use the top hand as the examining hand. If anything is there, chances are good that it will be found.

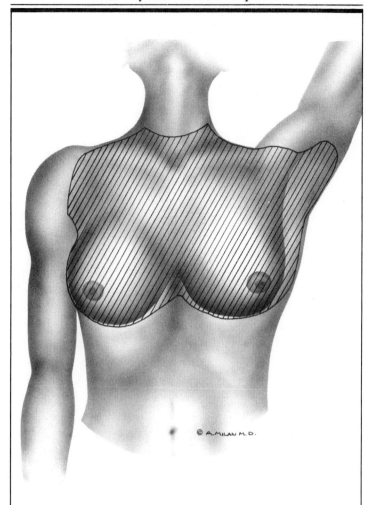

FIGURE 11. While our primary concern is with the breast proper, it is also necessary to examine the adjacent surrounding areas. Many people have accessory breast tissue that extends into the armpit, high on the chest wall or below the shelving margin on the chest. Lymph nodes may also be present in the armpits or in the neck. In order to be safe, one must be thorough. Examine the entire shaded area in this diagram.

is perhaps the most popular (see Fig. 12). The entire breast area is examined utilizing a series of circles, starting first at the outer perimeter.

The arm on the side being examined is raised and the hand placed on the back of the head or behind the neck. The opposite hand always examines the opposite breast. It is recommended that one start at the top of the breast in the twelve o'clock position. While gently pressing down on the skin, the fingertips are rolled around in multiple tiny circles, a half-inch or so in diameter, following a path around the outer rim of the entire breast. On completion of this path, the fingers are moved inward about two finger breadths closer to the nipple. A second, smaller circular path is followed, covering an area immediately inside the one just examined. Depending on size, an average of four or five passes may be necessary to cover the entire breast.

Some extra time should be spent examining the structures under the areola and nipple. Do not be alarmed by the fact that the breasts are more granular in this area. This is usually due to prominent terminal milk ducts, or ampullas (see Fig. 2). The ducts are usually quite slippery and movable.

After completing the circular pattern examination, place the palm of your hand under one breast as though it were a shelf for the breast to rest on (see Fig. 13). While supporting the breast with the bottom hand, systematically make small circular movements with the top hand until you have felt everything in the breast between both hands. Now allow the top hand to be the immobilizing hand and systematically examine the under surface of the breast.

The soft milk glands and cysts are more readily palpable in the supine position and seem to disappear in the upright posture. The hard fixed lumps, however, are felt equally well in both positions. Lumps that are situated deep in the breast structure and close to the chest wall may be missed in the supine position. Bimanual examination in the upright posture seems to be a more effective means of

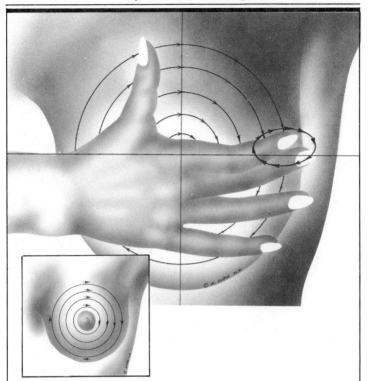

FIGURE 12. Utilizing the American Cancer Society's recommended concentric circle method, raise the arm of the side being examined above the head. Start to examine near the middle of the collarbone. Immobilize the skin with the fingertips, keeping the thumb extended. Roll the skin over the underlying breast tissue in small circular movements. Progress in a clockwise direction, making a multiple series of small circles as you advance around the outer rim of the breast. After a complete pattern is covered around the outer periphery of the breast, move the fingertips about two finger breadths closer to the center of the breast. Examine this second ring utilizing the same small circular movements. Continue to advance closer and closer to the nipple until the entire breast is examined. When you approach the nipple area, spend an extra moment because there often are a number of enlarged slippery milk glands and ducts at the rim of the areola. You should get to know these and know that they are there.

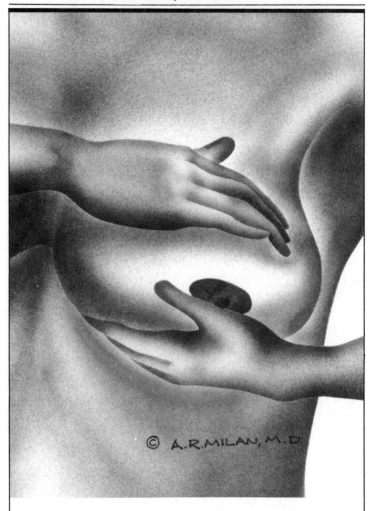

FIGURE 13. Using two hands can decrease the difficulty in examining large or pendulous breasts. One hand is placed beneath the breast and is used as a support. The other is utilized to examine the top surface of the breast. An effort is made to feel all the intervening tissue between the two hands. The procedure is then reversed so that the palm of the top hand is used as the support and the bottom hand is used to examine the under surface of the breast.

finding some of these. In any event, both methods are necessary in order to perform a thorough examination.

THE TWELVE-STROKE "CLOCK" METHOD

In my daily practice we use the "clock" method (see Fig. 14). This is a disciplined method and minimizes the possibility of "cutting corners." Following the twelve divisions of the clock allows little chance of missing anything. The procedure is performed by starting at the middle of the left collarbone. Raise the left arm above the head. Examine the left breast with the right hand. While immobilizing the skin with gentle pressure, move the tips of the fingers over the breast in small circular patterns progressing downward toward the center of the nipple. Then, with the same movements of the fingertips, proceed from the nipple upward to the "one o'clock" position. Move into the armpit to the "two o'clock" position and examine this area thoroughly. Proceed from the armpit in toward the nipple again. Then, from the nipple, palpate outward to "three o'clock," then in from "four o'clock," out to "five o'clock," etc., until the entire breast has been examined.

While it may take somewhat longer than other "systematic pattern" methods, I feel that the "clock" method is more thorough. If anything is there, the chance of finding it is much better with this disciplined and repetitive twelve-stroke procedure.

EXAMINATION WHILE LYING FLAT

The second portion of the breast self-examination is performed while lying flat in bed or on a couch (see Fig. 15). Some physicians have advocated that the palpation be carried out through a piece of fabric covering the breasts, e.g., a remnant of sheeting, a towel or a slip. This appears

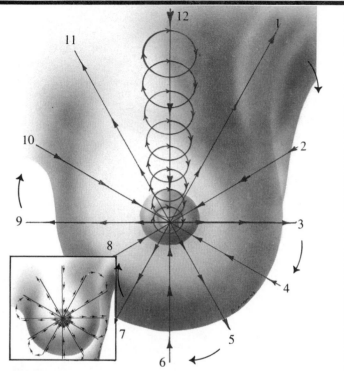

FIGURE 14. The method of palpation used with the circular pattern is also effective in covering the breast area on small breasts; however, a more regimented "route" is followed on the larger breasts. Start at the center of the collarbone (the twelve o'clock position of the left breast). Make small circular movements with the fingertips and advance downward toward the nipple. Advance outward from the nipple to the one o'clock position, then move into the armpit. Feel around in the armpit, then work your way around to the two o'clock position. From this point, proceed back inward toward the nipple area. From the nipple, move outward to three o'clock, then inward from four o'clock, etc., until a pass is made for every segment of the clock. Twelve passes are made to systematically cover the entire breast area. Spend some extra time around the nipple area before moving to the other breast. If you find something, check the same area in the other breast. If it has a mirror image in the other breast, it is less likely to be serious. If you are in doubt, have it checked by your doctor.

to assist in immobilizing the skin with the fingertips so that the deeper structures of the breast may be felt with greater facility. If the breasts are large, they will have a predisposition to fall to the side. It is advisable to place a pillow or several folded towels beneath the shoulder of the breast that is being examined (see Figs. 16 and 17). Raise the shoulder high enough so that the breast is centrally situated on top of the chest and does not fall either to the midline or to the armpit side. In this position, the chest wall will serve as a backstop, thereby improving the accuracy of the examination. The arm on the side being examined is raised and placed over the forehead or behind the head, whichever is more comfortable. Placing the arms in this position causes the large pectoral muscles, situated beneath the breast, to be moved out of the way toward the midline. The breast is first examined with the arm raised over the head. The examination is then repeated with the arm in a relaxed position at the side. Follow the details of either the circular pattern method or the twelve-stroke method described earlier in this chapter (see Figs. 12 and 14).

SOME POSSIBLE FINDINGS

AREAS OF THICKENING

In certain individuals who have heavy, pendulous breasts, or who have lost excessive weight, areas of benign thickening may be detected that could produce some apprehension. The angle at the junction of the under surface of the breast at its attachment to the chest wall can undergo a process of thickening due to fibrosis. This area is known as the "shelving margin." Not infrequently, a ropelike band may be felt in this region. Thickenings will usually be present in both breasts and will be approximately the same size and have the same degree of firmness. They are usually quite harmless, but there is no guarantee that a

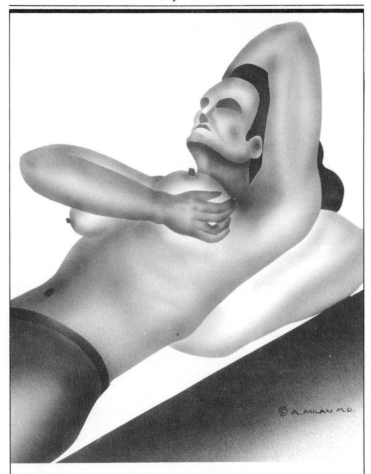

FIGURE 15. Lie flat on a bed or couch. Place a pillow or folded towels under the shoulder of the breast that is being examined so that the breast will be spread uniformly on the surface of the chest. The arm on the side of the breast being examined is placed either over the forehead or behind the head. This positioning moves the large chest muscles out of the way. The breast is examined by the hand from the opposite side, feeling with the flat surfaces of two or more fingertips. The arm is now placed comfortably at the side and the breast is reexamined in the same manner. The pillow is then placed under the other shoulder for examination of the opposite breast.

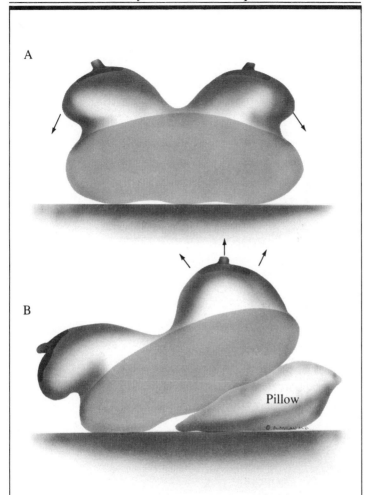

FIGURE 16. Large or pendulous breasts are difficult to examine because of their predisposition to fall to one side. This makes it difficult to feel anything in the lateral quadrants (A) with any degree of accuracy. A pillow is placed under the shoulder of the breast being examined so that the axis of the nipple points straight upward. The breast will flatten out nicely, producing a gently rounded contour (B). It is difficult to feel a breast mass unless it is backed up by the chest wall or the other hand, particularly if it is in the outer periphery of the breast.

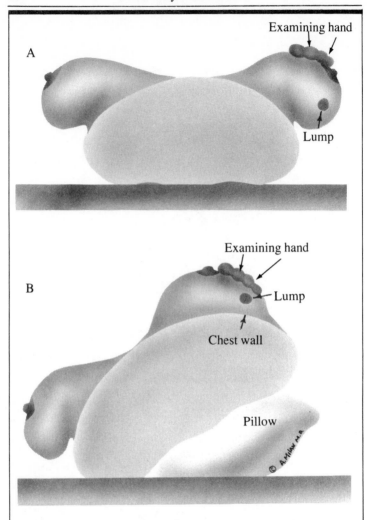

FIGURE 17. A lump is situated in the outer quadrant of the breast shown in this diagram. If the examining hand is on the front of the breast, pushing downward on the lump in the over-hanging area, chances are very good that this lump will be missed (A). If the shoulder is elevated with a pillow, the breast spreads uniformly over the chest wall and the lump is entrapped between the chest wall and the examining hand (B).

lump cannot develop in this area. Palpate thickenings carefully during each examination and be wary of any changes in them.

The second most common site of thickening is the upper outer quadrant of the breast (see Fig. 18). Thickening here is less likely to be serious in nature if it is identical in both breasts. The upper outer quadrant is the most frequent site of breast cancer. If a thickening is found in this area and it is only on one side, it should be checked by a physician. If thickenings are present, keep this area under surveillance for any change. At the slightest indication of abnormality, seek an evaluation from your physician.

MISCELLANEOUS HARMLESS LUMPS AND BUMPS

There are a multitude of miscellaneous harmless lumps and bumps that are capable of creating great anxiety when discovered during self-examination (see Fig. 19). It is a good practice to have your physician evaluate these "pseudo-lumps" and to be reassured that they are normal anatomical findings. Peace of mind will be well worth the time and effort expended.

JOINTS AND PROMINENCES. The framework of the chest wall has many bony prominences, joints and cartilage junctions of the rib cage that are commonly mistaken for breast lumps. The xiphoid bone is a small cartilaginous bone situated in the midline at the lower end of the breastbone. The xiphoid is frequently bent outward during pregnancy, and the sudden discovery of a hard "lump" produced by this bony prominence can cause concern. Similarly, the ends of unattached, or "floating," ribs can cause lumps or prominences on one or both sides of the chest.

ACCESSORY BREAST TISSUE. The configuration of the major part of the breast is hemispherical. Often, however, there is a tail of breast tissue extending up into the armpit and giving the breast a "comma" shape. There can be a

AREAS OF THICKENING

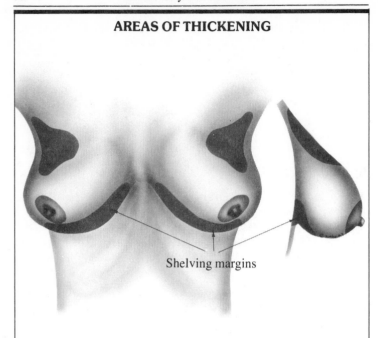

Shelving margins

FIGURE 18. In the woman with heavy breasts and particularly in the middle-aged and elderly woman, there are areas of dense fibrous depositions that are frequently mistaken for serious breast lumps. These are usually found to be mirror images in both breasts. A thick band of fibrous tissue is deposited in the lower rim of the breast at a point where it attaches to the chest wall. Usually firm and elongated, this is known as a ''thickening in the shelving margin.'' Though it is usually harmless, there is no guarantee that a tumor cannot start in this area. It should be carefully checked each month; if there is any change, consult your physician.

Another common area of thickening is the upper outer portions of the breast, as indicated by the dark area in the diagram. This again is thick fibrous tissue and is less worrisome if the exact mirror image is found in the other breast.

HARMLESS "LUMPS" COMMONLY MISTAKEN FOR SERIOUS BREAST LUMPS

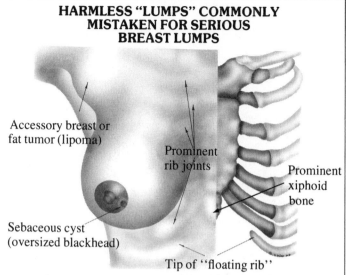

Accessory breast or fat tumor (lipoma)

Prominent rib joints

Prominent xiphoid bone

Sebaceous cyst (oversized blackhead)

Tip of "floating rib"

FIGURE 19. This illustration depicts some of the common pitfalls that alarm many women unnecessarily. The joints between the ribs, rib cartilages and breast bones frequently produce worrisome lumps and bumps under or near the breast.

The xiphoid bone is a small tail of bone situated exactly in the midline and is attached to the bottom of the breastbone. This may be angulated outward and not infrequently frightens people as an unknown lump.

One or more ribs, frequently referred to as "floating ribs," may be unattached to the bottom of the breastbone. Occasionally the tip of one of these ribs may be very prominent and can be misconstrued as a breast "lump."

Lipomas are fat tumors. It may be impossible to distinguish them from breast tissue. They are commonly found in the armpits but may occur anywhere on the surface of the body.

Sebaceous cysts are structures found in the skin proper. These are caused by a "stopped-up" oil gland, or sebaceous gland, and can range in size from a pinhead to a walnut. Since the areola surrounding the nipple contains many oil glands, it is a likely spot to find sebaceous cysts. The cysts usually have a tiny black dot or pore in their center. Since they are attached and are part of the skin itself, pinching or lifting the skin causes the sebaceous cysts to lift with it. They are one of the commonest of the harmless "attached" lumps.

considerable amount of breast tissue in the tail, complete with nipple, areola, ducts, etc. This accessory breast tissue may be found in either one armpit or both (see Figs. 19, 20, and 38). It can become swollen and tender with the menstrual period, with pregnancy and with lactation. Accessory breast tissue must receive the same attention in the breast self-examination as does the major portion of the breast since it is subject to the same pathology.

In our embryonic life, we have what is known as the "milk line" (see Fig. 20). This extends in a line from the armpit to the inside of the thighs. Frequently there are multiple nipples as well as accessory islands of breast tissue situated in this line. They may resemble pigmented moles, but when carefully inspected are found to be small nipples. Not infrequently, there is an accumulation of breast tissue in the armpit. It may present itself simply as a bulge of soft breast tissue or it may be complete with nipple and areola. This bulge is a frequent source of anxiety but is essentially an anatomical variant. It should feel exactly like the breast. Since it is breast tissue, it is vulnerable to the same pathology as the breast.

LIPOMAS. Certain individuals have a predisposition to make fatty tumors known as "lipomas." Lipomas may occur anywhere on the body and the breasts are no exception. Their consistency is very similar to that of normal breast tissue and it may be impossible to distinguish one from the other. They are usually harmless, but enlarging lipomas may be mistaken for certain breast tumors and it is advisable that they be kept under the surveillance of your physician.

SEBACEOUS CYSTS. Perhaps the most common of the intradermal (within-the-skin) lumps are the sebaceous cysts. These harmless lumps are overactive single oil glands that have become "stopped up." They can occur within the skin on any part of the body. The oily secretion accumulates within the gland and produces a hard, fixed

act mirror-image breasts is definitely in the minor-
ce most women have dissimilar breasts, it is ex-
important for each woman to familiarize herself
exact configuration of her breasts in their normal
he concern is not with how unalike they are, but
w they *change* from the pattern and appearance
ve been observed as normal. Any unexplainable
in appearance of one breast that is not similarly
ted in the other should automatically arouse one's
y and launch an investigation procedure as to why
occurred. Most breast cancers are situated within
ast proper, and therefore the most logical place for
cesses of distortion must originate here. As de-
earlier, the contour and silhouette of the breast
maintained by a lacelike mesh of delicate structural
nown as Cooper's ligaments. Since most breast
are adherent, they are very capable of distorting
licate meshwork, thereby producing a visible
in the configuration of the breast. The adhesive
of the cancer may cause further distortion by at-
nt to the skin, nipple or muscles of the chest wall.

ERVATION BEFORE A MIRROR

ctively carry out this part of the examination, a
irror with a good light placed off to the side is
l.(See Figs. 21 and 22.)

ARMS AT THE SIDES

rect in front of the mirror with both arms resting
at your sides. Carefully observe the relative size of
sts. Is one lower or higher than the other? Are the
round and smooth or are there dimples, indents,
ns or bulges that distort the outline? Do both nip-
nt outward (everted), or is one or both of them

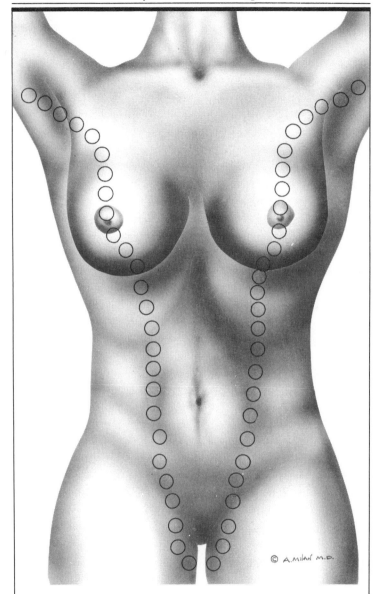

FIGURE 20. The "milk line," represented here by small circles, extends from the armpit to the pubic region. Any and all
components of breast tissue may by found along this line.

lump. A tiny sebaceous cyst is known to the layman as a "blackhead." Since the nipple areola has many oil glands in its periphery, sebaceous cysts are commonly found in the nipple area. They are "fixed lumps" and move with the skin since they are situated within the skin itself. If one observes carefully, a tiny pinpoint-sized black dot or dimple can be found in the center of most sebaceous cysts.

CHAPT
BREAST
EXAMINA
THE VIS
ASPE

In evaluating the mass of cl
"what brought the patient to
very top of the list that it w
physician, however, may repor
as a dimple, indentation, skin
sion, as his first finding. Not in
these signs long before the tum
duce a lump that is discernible t

Regrettably, the powers of
ascribed the same degree of i
examination as has the sense c
feeling for a lump is all there is t
need only be reminded that by t
ered, the cancer may already ha

Not only my personal op
teaches that many telltale signs
before an actual lump can be fel
of this critical visual exam has
extremely early cancers, often t
pated.

Contrary to the belief of m

with ex
ity. Sir
tremely
with th
state. T
with h
that ha
change
duplica
curiosi
this has
the bre
the pro
scribed
form is
fibers k
cancers
this de
change
quality
tachme

OBS

To effe
large n
essenti

Stand e
loosely
the bre
contou
retracti
ples po

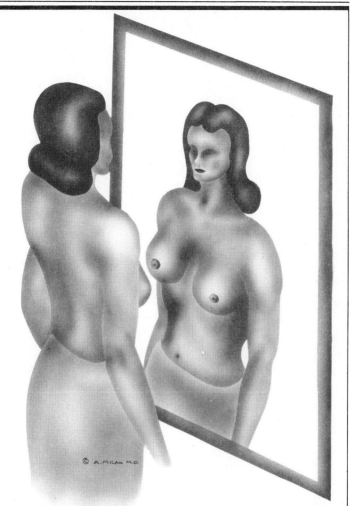

FIGURE 21. Stand before a large mirror with your arms in a relaxed position at your sides. Place a lamp off to one side. Inspect carefully to learn what is normal for you. On each subsequent examination, concentrate on *changes* that were not noted on earlier examinations. Look for distortion, dimpling, indentation, contour changes, bulging, nipple inversions, etc., that were not present on your previous examination. Inspect carefully while standing still, then while turning from side to side.

UPRIGHT POSITION, RELAXED

Elbows back

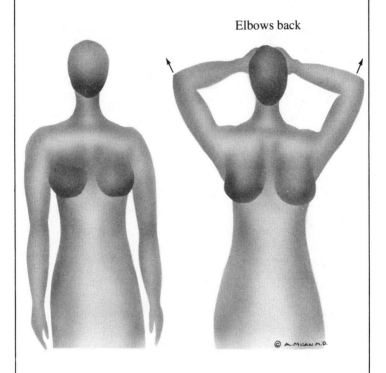

FIGURE 22. Examination before a mirror is first carried out with the arms relaxed at either side. Then the body is turned slowly from side to side. Look for dimples, indentations, retractions, distortions and skin changes. Place the hands behind the head, push the elbows backward and inspect again. This tightens the skin and may reveal subtle changes.

turned "outside in" (inverted)? Are there any fissures or clefts in the nipples? What is the comparative size of the areolas (pigmented halo of skin surrounding the nipple)? Inspect the skin of the breast carefully to determine if there is anything unusual about its texture. Dermatological conditions like psoriasis, eczema, moles, rashes, etc., can involve the skin of the breasts just as they can any other part of the body. You must be aware of what is normal for you; otherwise there is no way for you to detect subtle but significant changes.

After you have carefully inspected the breasts for the above criteria, slowly turn from side to side, first bringing one breast forward and then the other. Allowing the light to cast shadows on the breast helps point out any bulges, retractions, dimples or distortions.

At this point, it is important to recollect from your medical history factors that may have been responsible for changes in symmetry or configuration. These factors may include surgery, infection, injury or overuse of one arm (tennis, bowling, etc).

"LOOK-ALIKES"

There are many harmless conditions that may exhibit all of the outward appearances of a serious problem. A flying ant or a termite? A harmless or poisonous snake? Differentiation may require the skills of an expert. Certain harmless "look-alikes" pertaining to the breasts are listed below to help clarify and recognize their benign nature.

1. NIPPLE SECRETIONS (*Fig. 23*). Try to express some secretion from the nipples by gently pressing with the sides of the fingers. If secretion can be expressed from both nipples, it is probably hormonal in origin. Nipple secretion is a common occurrence. It may be white, yellow, brown or bloody. Secretion is especially common following a pregnancy and may last even years if the proper supporting

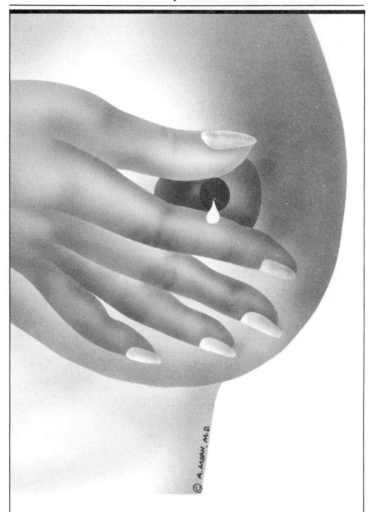

FIGURE 23. Gently try to express some secretion from the nipples. Nipple secretion is a common and often harmless finding. If it is present on both sides, it is probably hormonal in origin. Secretion is common particularly after a pregnancy. Secretions that occur spontaneously are of more significance than those produced by forceful expression. Make it a habit to inspect your bra every day. Persistent nipple discharge or bleeding should be investigated by your physician.

garments were not worn. It may also occur in the patient who has recently stopped using birth-control pills. Make it a habit to inspect your bra for nipple bleeding or discharge when you undress. If the bleeding or discharge is persistent, it should be evaluated by your physician.

2. INVERTED NIPPLES (*Fig. 24*). An inverted nipple is one that is turned "outside in." It may have been inverted since birth and never came out. Or it may be everted part of the time but usually turns inward again. There are varying degrees of inversion. While some nipples are just about flat, others may be markedly inverted. If the inversion has been present for a long time, it probably has little significance. What is significant, however, is a *change*. A nipple that has always been everted and then suddenly becomes inverted represents an important change and should be investigated. "Significant change" must be differentiated from "serious change" because there are certain harmless conditions that can produce not only nipple inversion but other associated visual changes.

3. NIPPLE SORES AND ULCERS (*Fig. 25*). Inspect for sores, ulcerated area or eczema involving the nipple and/or areola. An ulcer on the nipple or areola that has been present for more than two weeks and that does not appear to be healing should be checked by your physician, as should any other bothersome skin condition of the nipples.

4. DISTORTION OF THE NIPPLE AXIS. If you were to draw an imaginary line through the center of the nipple in the direction in which the nipple points, this would be considered the nipple "axis." This axis is usually different for both breasts. Does one nipple point off to the side, upward, downward or inward? It is important to know what is normal for you. Any deviation from the preexisting axis may indicate a significant change.

5. DIMPLES, INDENTS, RETRACTIONS OF THE NIPPLE OR AREOLA. Many people have symmetrical or mirror-

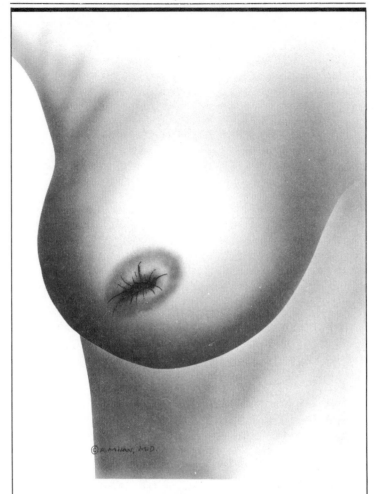

FIGURE 24. Inversion of the nipple means that the nipple is turned "outside in." This may be perfectly normal and may have been present since birth or may have come about from an injury, from surgery, from an infection or from excessive weight gain. If it has always been "out," or everted, and only recently turned inward, or if it is out when in the upright position but inverts on leaning forward and this condition was not present before, it must be evaluated by your physician. Again, *change* is the key word. The cause may be entirely harmless; nevertheless, it may not be and must therefore be evaluated.

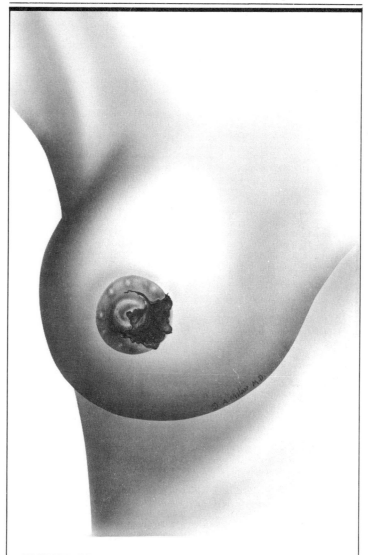

FIGURE 25. A persistent ulcer anywhere on the body, particularly one that refuses to heal, should be checked by your physician. Again there are a multitude of harmless skin conditions to explain the findings. Only your physician is qualified to tell you if the ulcer is benign in nature or if it requires further investigation.

image dimples in both breasts within the pigmented area of the areola. These dimples are usually situated to the lateral side of or just below the nipple. They are a difficult sign to interpret, particularly with the aging processes. It is more significant if only one breast is involved and if the dimple represents a recent change.

FACTORS RELATED TO THE SKIN

1. "ORANGE PEEL SKIN" *(Fig. 26)*. Whenever a lymph duct draining a certain area of skin is blocked, the lymph fluid backs up and makes what in appearance would resemble a giant mosquito bite or hive. The skin becomes raised, shiny and firm. The pores are enlarged, become deeper and are spread further apart. This finding has been aptly named "orange peel skin" and on the breast may be caused by infections involving the arm and armpits, as well as by insect bites. Since this type of swelling in the breast can also accompany certain types of tumor growths, the presence of this sign warrants immediate attention.

2. PATCHES OF REDNESS. Your attention should be directed to any isolated area of redness and blushing on the skin. This may be a sign of inflammation or infection, particularly if the area is warm and tender. It may also be associated with an increase in blood supply for any number of reasons. If it persists, the problem should be evaluated by your physician.

3. PROMINENT BLOOD VESSEL PATTERN. The woman who has had a pregnancy is quite familiar with the enlargement, tenderness, warmth and increased blood vessel pattern of the breasts. At times, the pattern may take on the appearance of a road map tattooed upon the breast surfaces. Birth-control pills and other hormones are capable of producing the same picture. The breast veins normally become engorged in the last two weeks of the menstrual cycle. Prominent breast veins may also be a sign of underlying diseases of the chest wall or blood vessels. If the

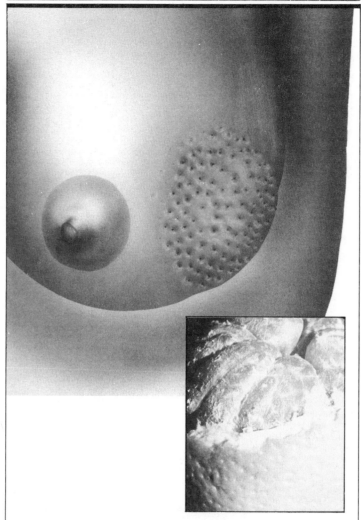

FIGURE 26. Raised, smooth, shiny areas of skin with widely separated and deep pores are signs of blocked superficial lymph channels. This finding may occur with many infections that may be local in origin or may involve the armpit. It can also occur from insect bites. Since it is nevertheless a sign associated with certain tumors, it must be evaluated by your physician. A partially peeled orange is shown to reveal the derivation of the name "orange peel skin."

veins of one breast have become more prominent than those of the other, and if this sign had not been present in the past, the condition should be evaluated.

4. SKIN ULCERS ON THE BREASTS. Persistent areas of ulceration involving the skin of the breast are evaluated in the same manner as nipple ulcers and should be examined by your physician.

5. MOLES AND FRECKLES (*Fig. 27*). Moles, freckles and similar skin conditions can involve the breasts just as they can the skin on any other part of the body. Worry about them as much as you would about moles anywhere else on your body. Malignant moles can be just as vicious as any other cancer. While we are alerted to look for changes in size, color, consistency or halo formation in any existing moles, it is my opinion that these changes should not be given the chance to occur. If there are raised, smooth, wide-based pigmented moles anywhere on the body, and particularly at sites where they are likely to be injured, it is better to have them removed. If we wait for them to change, we are simply waiting for cancer to happen. Raised, flat-surfaced, pigmented moles situated on or around the bra strap line, necklace line, belt line or hairbrush line are potential time bombs. The priority for removal of moles from these sites should be high.

RELATIVE SIZE AND SHAPE OF THE BREASTS

1. NORMAL ASYMMETRY. It is important to remember that most individuals have unalike breasts. It is equally important to remember that our primary interest is not in normal asymmetry, but rather in a *change* from the preexisting normal status. One must carefully define any and all normal differences between the two breasts and either record or remember these patterns in all future examinations.

2. NIPPLE PLACEMENT. Are the nipples and areolas situ-

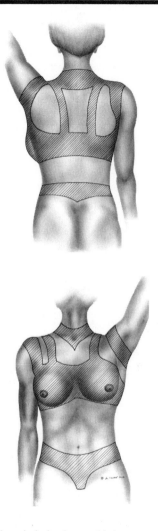

FIGURE 27. Chronic irritation and injury to certain pigmented moles may cause them to undergo cancerous transformation. The shaded areas in these diagrams are sites of particular vulnerability. These include the necklace line, the sleeve line, the bra strap line, the surface of the breasts and the belt line. It is advisable to have all suspicious-looking moles removed, particularly those situated in the hazardous areas noted here.

ated in the same location as during previous examinations? Does one appear to be lower, higher, turned upward or downward, inward or outward? Again, a *change* from the original pattern is of utmost concern.

3. SIZE OF BREASTS. Has there been any change in size? Has one breast become disproportionately larger or smaller than previously? Allow for weight loss or gain, pregnancy, surgery or asymmetric exercises.

4. CONTOUR CHANGES. Examine the contours carefully for change, particularly while turning from side to side. Look for areas of flattening, bulging, indentation, dimpling or retraction. Has any distortion of the overall shape altered the breast from its previous configuration? Emphasis is on *change*.

ARMS RAISED

After a careful inspection for the preceding criteria has been carried out with the arms at the sides, a similar ritual of observation is performed with the arms in other positions. Again, it is our motive to capitalize on the ability of the tumor to adhere to the skin, the chest wall or the Cooper's ligaments within the breast. Changing the position of the arms can tighten the skin overlying the breasts as well as alter the position of the underlying pectoral muscles. If a small breast tumor is attached to the muscles of the chest wall, it will not permit this portion of the breast to move as readily as the unaffected portion. A telltale dimple, retraction or bulge is thus produced on the surface of the breast when the position of the breast is altered. Changing the position of the arms or allowing the breasts to hang downward by leaning forward are the most effective ways of detecting these changes. With each change in position of the arms, the breasts are inspected first while facing the mirror directly, then by turning the body slowly from side to side. The side lighting casts a shadow that helps to identify any existing irregularity.

TOP VIEW

Light
→

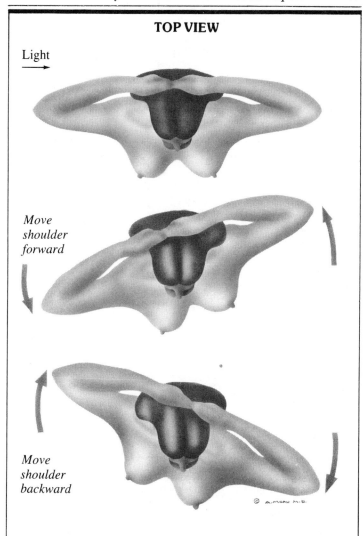

*Move
shoulder
forward*

*Move
shoulder
backward*

FIGURE 28. Inspection before the mirror with the hands clasped behind the head is carried out first while facing the mirror directly, then while slowly turning from side to side. The light, which is off to the side, will produce brighter spots and shadows on the breasts and help to disclose dimples, indentations and distortions that may not have been previously noted. This diagram was made while looking down from above.

HANDS CLASPED BEHIND HEAD

The arms are now raised and the hands clasped behind the head (see Fig. 28). The elbows are pushed backward so that the skin over the breasts will be stretched. The body is turned from side to side as previously and the criteria described earlier are noted.

PECTORAL CONTRACTION MANEUVERS

The hands are now placed in front of the forehead with palms clasped together (see Fig 29). Squeeze and hold the hands together firmly so that the large chest muscles are tightened. This maneuver raises the breasts and tightens the skin, thus bringing out any underlying dimples or retractions that might be present.

When performing the pectoral contraction maneuvers, the overweight individual may detect some small "fat dimples" in the breasts. These are not abnormal and usually occur on the lateral and under surfaces of the breasts. They are particularly common in areas of old stretch marks. If they appear equal in size and are in the same position in both breasts, they are probably due to subcutaneous fat. If there is pronounced dimpling or retraction of the skin involving only one breast and there is no previous medical or surgical history to explain it, a physician should be consulted.

The second pectoral contraction maneuver is performed by placing both palms flat on the sides of the hips and squeezing firmly downward. The same observations are made as above while facing the mirror directly and while turning from side to side.

LEANING FORWARD POSITION

The leaning forward position holds the greatest potential for accentuating the normal as well as the abnormal variables (see Fig. 30). I feel that this position is the most productive of all the observation tests and gives us the

PECTORAL CONTRACTION MANEUVERS

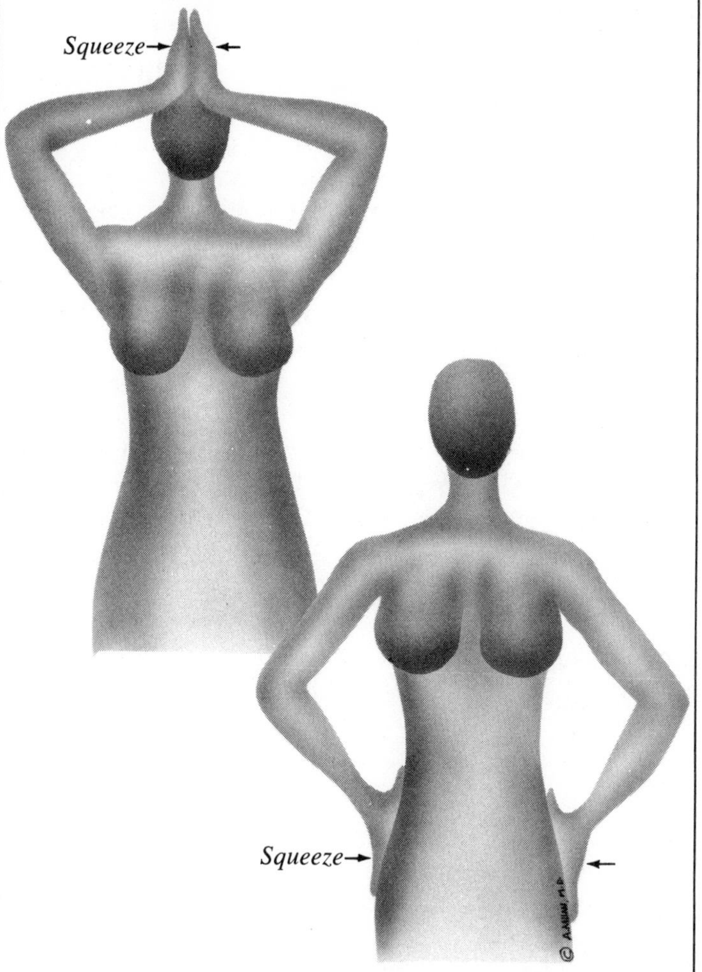

Squeeze→   *←*

Squeeze→   *←*

FIGURE 29. Place the palms together in front of the forehead and squeeze them together. This maneuver tightens the pectoral muscles. If there is a scar or growth which attaches the breast to these muscles, a dimple or distortion may be produced. Inspect while turning from side to side. Now place hands on hips and squeeze downward firmly. Inspect first while facing mirror directly, then turn from side to side.

greatest hope for early detection of existing problems.

As described earlier, the shape or form of the breast is maintained by the presence of Cooper's ligaments attached to the under surface of the skin and to the chest wall. Any new process within the breast that may be attached to these fibers has the capability of shortening or distorting them. When these fibers become entangled in an old scar or in a new growth, an unyielding band may be formed that binds the skin to the underlying chest muscles. When one leans forward, the normal breast structure will fall away, leaving a dimple or distortion in the entangled area.

It is desirable to lean forward bending at the hips so that the breasts hang straight downward. This, of course, is performed before a large mirror. The arms may be held out straight or supported on the knees, backs of chairs or other objects. Whatever procedure is used, it should be carried out in the same manner each time.

LEANING FORWARD POSITION

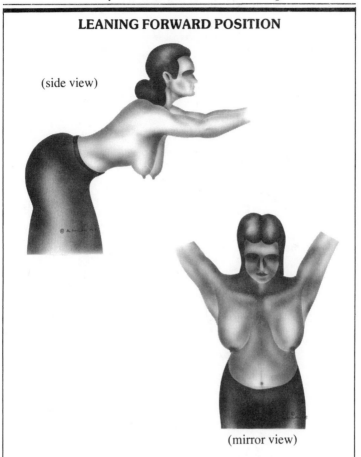

(side view)

(mirror view)

FIGURE 30. Lean forward in such a way that the breasts will point straight downward. It is better to flex at the hips rather than to "hunch over." The arms may be either held out straight or supported on the knees or a nearby object such as a chair back. Place a light off to one side.

This position may greatly accentuate existing breast asymmetry. Not invariably, one breast will be larger, smaller, pointier, rounder, flatter, etc. Carefully inspect the contour, size, nipple axis and distortion. Observe what is normal for you and remember what these variants are. The variants should cause little or no concern; however, a *change* from the existing pattern can be very important.

NORMAL VARIANTS
(leaning forward position)

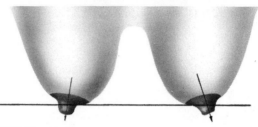

FIGURE 31. Women with breasts that are an exact mirror image of each other constitute a minority. There is almost always some variation in size, shape, contour, nipple axis, nipple shape, areolar size, etc. This is a diagram of breasts that are alike.

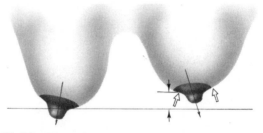

FIGURE 32. The left breast in this diagram is somewhat smaller. The contours and shapes are similar. The left nipple is higher than the right. The left nipple axis deviates laterally.

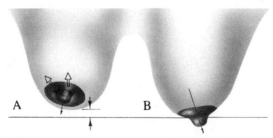

FIGURE 33. The right breast is higher and appears to be smaller. The entire areola is visible on the right, while only part of the left is apparent from this view. The right nipple axis is turned forward. The side view of this breast is depicted in Fig. 40B.

NORMAL VARIANTS
(leaning forward position)

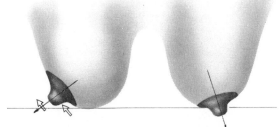

FIGURE 34. The right nipple axis deviates outward to the right side. Breasts are comparable in size. Contours are round and smooth.

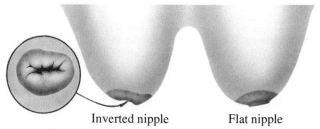

Inverted nipple   Flat nipple

FIGURE 35. The left nipple is almost flat, while the right is inverted. Neither of these findings is necessarily abnormal if it has been present for a long time or if it followed surgery or a breast infection. As a recent occurrence, its significance should be investigated.

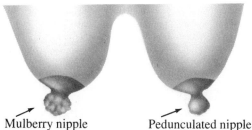

Mulberry nipple   Pedunculated nipple

FIGURE 36. The sizes and shapes of nipples may be as variable as people's faces. Occasionally, the nipple is found to be lobulated, with its surface resembling a mulberry; this is not abnormal. The pedunculated, or teardrop-shaped, nipple is a frequent normal variant.

NORMAL VARIANTS
(leaning forward position)

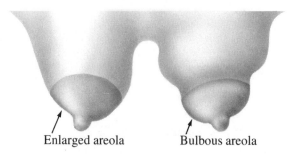

Enlarged areola   Bulbous areola

FIGURE 37. The pigmented halo, or areola, that surrounds the nipple may be variable in color and size. It may vary from a pale pink to black. It may be very small or it may cover half the breast and still be normal.

If the pigmented areola bulges above the surface of the breast proper, it is called a bulbous areola and is not abnormal.

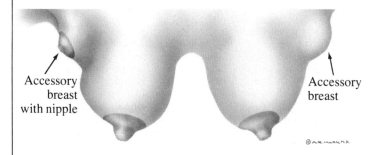

Accessory
breast
with nipple

Accessory
breast

FIGURE 38. Many individuals have what they take to be large folds of fat in the forward portion of their armpits. Careful examination of these "fat pockets" will impart the same sensation as will the main breast tissue. They may be either a tail of breast tissue extending into the armpit or an accessory breast. There may or may not be a nipple. This is not abnormal.

NORMAL VARIANTS
(leaning forward position)

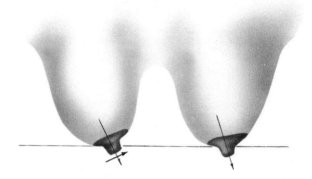

FIGURE 39. Breasts are the same size. Right nipple axis deviates inward.

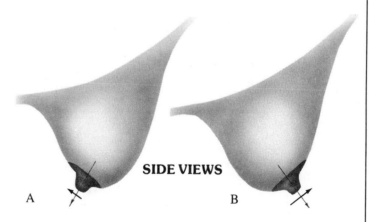

SIDE VIEWS

A

B

FIGURE 40. Diagram A shows the nipple axis turned downward so that the nipple would not be seen in the leaning forward position. In diagram B, the nipple axis is turned upward. This is the same as seen in the front view in Fig. 33A. These are normal variants if they have always turned in this manner.

POSSIBLE ABNORMALITIES

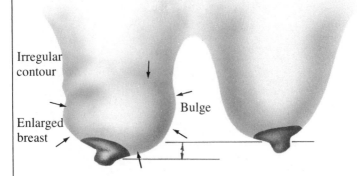

Irregular
contour

Enlarged
breast

Bulge

FIGURE 41. Assuming that both breasts shown here were once comparable in size and shape, the right breast appears to have enlarged. The entire right breast hangs lower. There is a distinct bulge on the inner and front surface of the breast. The right nipple axis deviates laterally. The lateral side of the right breast has a distinct change in contour, with varying bulges and shadows.

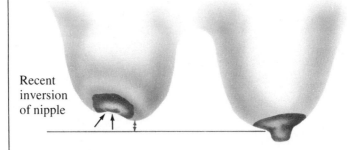

Recent
inversion
of nipple

FIGURE 42. Nipple inversion can be significant when it is a recent occurrence. If the nipple is everted in the upright position but inverted in the leaning forward maneuver, or if it had always been everted then gradually became inverted, the cause must be determined. Relatively harmless conditions like fatty degeneration, infection or swelling of the terminal milk ducts may give a benign reason for the finding; however, a possible tumor must be ruled out.

POSSIBLE ABNORMALITIES

Breast
elevated

Retraction→

Nipple axis
rotated out

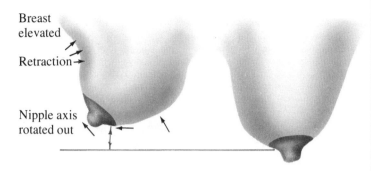

FIGURE 43. A distinct indentation is noted in the lateral side of the right breast. Associated with this indentation is a ridge and shadow on the front part of the breast. The entire breast is lifted higher and the nipple axis deviates to the side. If this represents a change that cannot be explained, it is significant and must be investigated.

Breast
elevated

Indentation
(dimpling)

Nipple
axis
upward

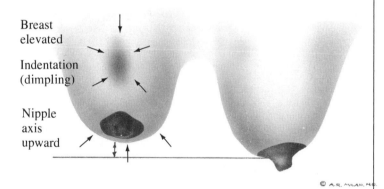

© A.R. MILAN. M.D.

FIGURE 44. A shadow is noted on the forward surface of the right breast. The entire breast is higher and the nipple is turned upward. If this represents a change from the previous status and there is no explanation for its cause, it must be investigated.

POSSIBLE ABNORMALITIES

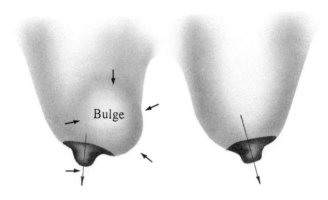

FIGURE 45. The size and shape of the right breast has changed. A bulge has formed on the inner forward surface, which in turn has caused the nipple axis to turn inward. This drawing was made from the breast of a young woman who reported a bulge of sudden onset. The surface of the bulge was smooth, slippery and unattached. The diagnosis of a cyst was made. A half-ounce of fluid was aspirated and the bulge disappeared. A similar picture could occur with a broken blood vessel, breast abscess or milk cyst (galactocoele) in a nursing mother. Needless to say, it could also be a tumor.

THE MECHANICS OF CHANGE

The exact interpretation of certain findings detected on breast examination may be very elusive. Agonizing decisions between watchful waiting and surgical intervention may become exceedingly difficult for both patient and physician. In light of the nature of our enemy and the fact that it never gives us a break, it is my opinion that if mistakes are to be made they should be made on the safe side. I would much prefer to have the opinion of a good pathologist rather than a good surgeon. Look-alikes on outward inspection of the breast may be carbon copies, yet one may be completely benign and the other malignant. The final answer must come from the pathologist, from what he observes under his microscope.

Each of the findings in the following series of illustrations could occur in a completely harmless situation or could have a malignant etiology. Whenever the slightest shadow of a doubt exists, I feel that it is best to consider the finding malignant until proven otherwise, and then to move heaven and earth to prove it benign.

The significance of Cooper's ligaments in maintaining the shape and form of the breast has been described. Indeed, the majority of the visual clues depend heavily on the integrity of these tiny ligaments. When some event, be it infection, injury, surgery or new growth, has occurred to produce ''entanglement'' of these intrinsic fibers, the disarray will cause some form of distortion or change from the usual form.

UPRIGHT POSITION

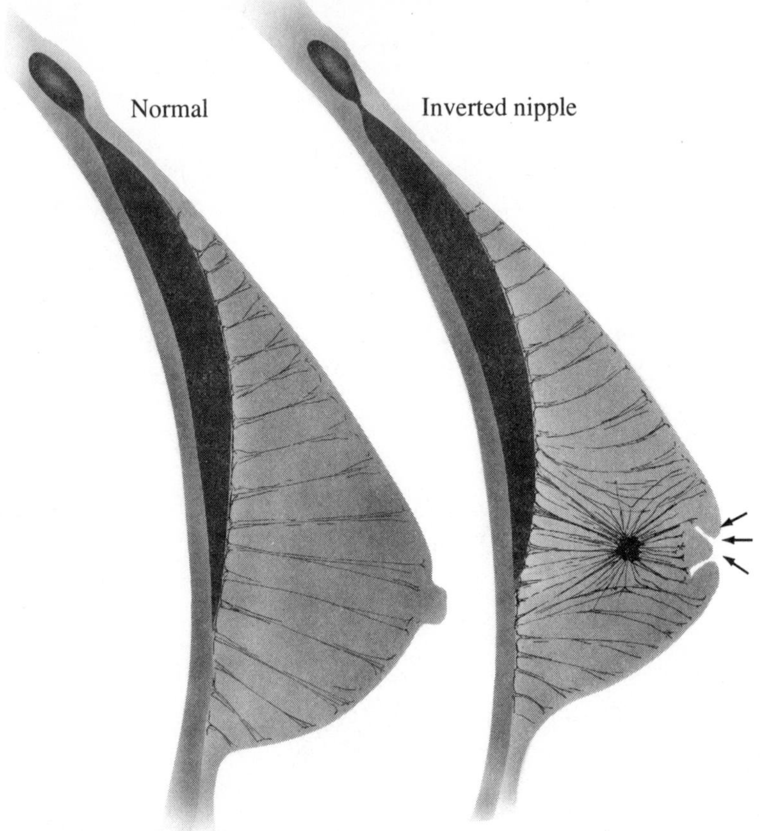

Normal   Inverted nipple

FIGURE 46. NIPPLE INVERSION: Nipple inversion is a relatively frequent finding in harmless as well as harmful situations. What is depicted here as a lump could just as well be an old mastitis, abscess or surgical scar. It could also be an organized blood clot or fat degeneration following an injury. A cross-sectional diagram of a normal breast in the upright position shows the normal partition fibers, or Cooper's ligaments. A small growth is portrayed behind the nipple, which has become entangled in the Cooper's ligaments of this area. The arrows in the upright position show how the nipple has been flattened, then drawn inward. The fixed ligaments now firmly anchor the nipple to the chest wall. In the leaning forward position, the unaffected portion of the breast falls away as it naturally would,

LEANING FORWARD POSITION

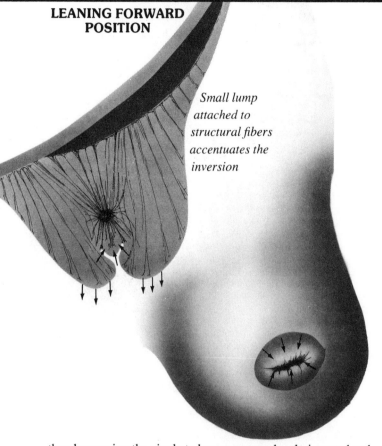

Small lump attached to structural fibers accentuates the inversion

thereby causing the nipple to become more deeply inverted and accentuating the sign of nipple retraction.

If the nipple is inverted *only* in the leaning forward position, *not* in the upright position, a problem may exist and your physician should be consulted. If the nipple has *always* been inverted while in the upright position, and does not invert deeper while leaning forward, this is probably an anatomical variant. Check with your doctor whenever there are doubts.

The harmless inversion is usually indistinguishable from the harmful. The history of change might help us since there are many benign explanations for this phenomenon, even if it is recent. In some instances, procedures may be necessary to clarify the diagnosis.

UPRIGHT POSITION   **LEANING FORWARD POSITION**

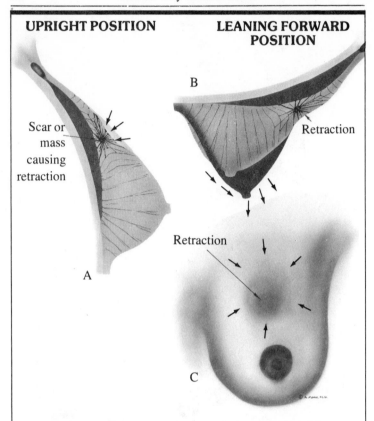

Scar or mass causing retraction

Retraction

A

B

Retraction

C

FIGURE 47. RETRACTION IN UPPER PORTION OF BREAST: Here we have another worrisome picture. In this case, residual scarring within the breast substance, resulting from a large abscess many years previously, produced the distortion. In the upright position (A) we see how the Cooper's ligaments have become entangled, effecting a retraction of the upper surface of the breast. Since these fibers have caused the overlying skin of the breast to remain attached to the chest wall, the leaning forward position (B) accentuates the indentation.

Similarly, the attachment will alter the nipple axis and cause it to deflect upward in the leaning forward position. Diagram C shows the image seen in the mirror. From outward appearances, it is impossible to differentiate this harmless indentation from a more serious condition. The assistance of a pathological evaluation is mandatory.

UPRIGHT POSITION   **LEANING FORWARD POSITION**

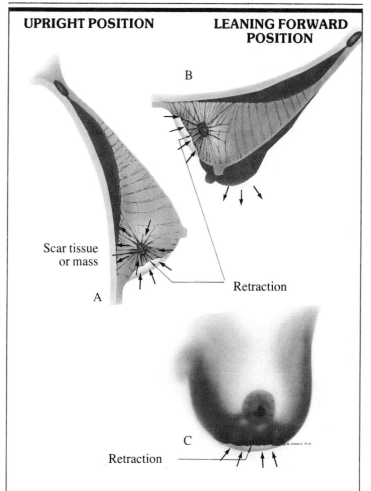

B

Scar tissue
or mass

A

Retraction

C

Retraction

FIGURE 48. RETRACTION IN LOWER PORTION OF BREAST: A similar picture of distortion is produced by the entanglement of Cooper's ligaments in the lower portion of the breast (A). In the leaning forward position (B) the upper portion of the breast is allowed to fall downward. The entanglement fixes the lower portion of the breast to the chest wall and causes the nipple axis to bend downward. The mirror view (C) reveals a flattened or indented crinkled appearance on the under surface of the breast.

CHAPTER 5
REACTIONS TO UNUSUAL FINDINGS

The fundamental purpose of this book is to underline those findings that will help us understand and appreciate all the early detection clues so as to improve the chances for long-term survival. But what is our course of action if a tiny area of suspicion has been discovered?

It is most disheartening to learn that a period of five to six months is the average amount of time that elapses between the moment the patient first discovers her problem and her first visit to the doctor. This is more than the amount of time needed to move her from the group of patients with an 80 to 90 percent chance of long-term cure to the group with a 40 percent or less chance of cure. Delay not only lessens the chances for survival but also wipes out many of the chances for reconstructive surgery.

A suspicious finding initiates the first shock wave, which poses the grave threat of the loss of an important sex symbol and its many associated emotional ramifications. The second shock wave ushers in a more awesome reality, namely, the threat to life itself. Emotionally, it is a most difficult task to wrestle with either of these situations. A major role in the ultimate outcome of breast cancer weighs heavily upon how each individual copes with these reactions. We are now confronted with the second and perhaps the most serious problem in this domain: delay and failure to act when the chances of cure are most favorable.

Why do people wait? The greatest common denominator is fear. Fear is responsible for converting many potentially curable situations into incurable ones. There is no simple way to overcome this emotion. The greatest weapons in conquering fear are probably dependent on how much faith an individual is able to muster: faith in herself, in her family and friends, in her physician, in her Creator. Closely akin to faith is knowledge. The patient must have an understanding of herself and her possible condition. She must be aware that the worrisome clues may be harmless in 70 to 80 percent of the cases; that if her problem is the worst, but is in an early stage, her chances of cure are excellent; that new breakthroughs happen daily but are dependent upon early detection and treatment; that many, many thousands of women have been successfully treated and cured, and have been capable of living a full and fruitful life; that she has a real friend in her physician, who shares her anxieties, will accept any and all challenges posed by her condition and stands ready to advise her and to help her in any way humanly possible.

Other reasons for delay are frequently given. When examined critically, however, these may be earth-shaking at the time but are rarely worth a delay that places the individual's life in jeopardy. It is better for the individual to "look out for number one" instead of worrying about the problems of others. In the long run, both the individual and the family will be better off.

A common reason given by many women for delay in seeking treatment is the fear of an unpredictable emotional response from the husband. This apprehension is often unwarranted, as the following anecdote will illustrate. A surgeon was counseling a patient and her husband on the nature of the lump he had found in the woman's breast. He explained the possibilities and the various courses of action he might take in the event of certain findings. During the conversation, the patient confessed her doubts as to how her husband would feel toward her following the surgery. The husband interrupted and resolved the problem deftly by stating: "Lady, I want you to know here and now that I am not married to your left boob; it is you I'm married to, it is you I love, and it is your life that is more precious to me than either or both of them." I feel that when the chips are really down, this would be the response of the average devoted American male.

The folks who make up the hard core of the group known as "rugged individualists," and who have never been seriously ill, assume a negativistic attitude. They feel that they are invincible and immune to the frailties of the human race and that "it can't happen to me." They will dispel the problem of a palpable breast lump from their minds until it is too late.

Shyness, false modesty and a cloistered life may be other factors in an unreasonable delay. Breast cancer is somewhat more common in the celibate woman and in those who have not borne children. Failure to perform breast self-examination, as well as failure to obtain periodic physical examinations, places these individuals at a higher risk.

Self-sacrifice or martyrdom, for want of a better term, may be another cause for delay. Women will refuse to divulge their secret finding because they do not want to spoil the plans for their child's wedding or their husband's new job. They do not want to upset a parent who has a terminal illness or a husband who had a recent heart attack. Often they will delay six months to a year, which not only may cost them their lives but may also cause the husband to have another heart attack. The individual should always consult the physician first, lay the facts on the line and let him be the adviser. The secretive delay can most assuredly end in unnecessary tragedy for many.

CHAPTER 6
BREAST SCREENING

O ur emphasis on improving the modalities of early detection becomes an exercise in futility if we do not immediately act upon the presence of a relevant clue. What is the course of action if a tiny area of suspicion has been discovered?

MAMMOGRAPHY

It is the firm opinion of the author that the most valuable diagnostic procedure developed in the war against cancer during this past century is x-ray mammography, or xero-mammography.

Despite the vast morass of controversy and irresponsible criticism of the mammogram, this procedure still excels as one of our most valuable and precise diagnostic tools. It is highly unlikely that the antagonists in this controversy would refuse to allow their wives to have mammography, if, indeed, a suspicious indentation, dimple or retraction had to be evaluated and surgery was the only other choice. The procedure can detect problems that cannot be uncovered by palpation or visual examination.

Mammography is not one hundred percent right all of the time, but in skillful hands it comes close. It is imperative that no x-ray procedure be abused or used without proper indication or respect. Some aspects of x-ray exposure have a cumulative effect. Though very small and often theoretical, these cumulative effects of diagnostic x-ray can be harmful. Resistance to ordering x-ray should increase in proportion to the total number of exposures to any type of x-ray the patient has had in the past. The request for mammography to clarify a suspicious finding remains a judgment call on the part of the physician. The heated emotionalism espoused by the lay press should not enter into life-threatening decision making. Complacency and delay may mute the chances of a cure for an early localized and curable malignancy. I personally would rather take my chances with the x-ray.

Weighing the benefits against the risks in mammographic screening, I feel that the woman at high risk of breast cancer should have a baseline mammogram to be used for future comparisons. The age for the first mammogram would have to be individualized according to the degree of risk as well as the physical findings. The next one may not be necessary for two, three, four or even five years, depending on how much the patient is at risk, what she finds during self-examination and what the physician discovers during his examinations. This investment may be of tremendous value if, five years into the future, a potential problem is detected and a repeat mammogram reveals no significant interval change from the initial picture. Surgery may be avoided and everyone will sleep a lot better. It is generally conceded, with essentially no controversy, that women over fifty years of age should have periodic mammography.

Modern technology has made vast strides in reducing the amount of irradiation received in the average mammogram to a fraction of what it was just a few years ago. Exceedingly high priorities in radiological research have been established to reduce the dosage even further so that this extremely valuable procedure may be used with even less apprehension.

A brief explanation is in order so that the reasons for the existing controversy may be better understood by all. The standard unit used to measure the amount of radiation exposure is called the "roentgen" or the "rad." There is a great difference between the amount of radiation energy emitted by the source of exposure and the precise amount of x-ray energy actually absorbed. A multitude of factors may intercede to produce a great variance between the amount of irradiation emitted and the amount actually absorbed by the individual. The difference between x-ray exposure and x-ray absorption may be more clearly understood if we compare the difference between simply being out of doors in the summer sun (exposure) and the actual sunburn received (absorbed energy).

Much of the current controversy and fear linking x-ray to cancer is derived from two reports that appeared in 1965 and 1968. The first concerned a group of tuberculosis patients who had been treated for their disease by lung collapse (pneumothorax) therapy. It was mandatory that this procedure, performed two or three times a week for a period of one or two years, be carried out under direct fluoroscopic visualization. The equipment and techniques used at that time (fifteen to forty years ago) delivered a dosage of radiation ten to twenty times greater than our modern technology. In the women thus exposed, there was a higher incidence of breast cancer than in the average citizen. It is estimated that each exposure was approximately 20 rads of irradiation to each breast. Our modern mammography units are calibrated to deliver approximately ⅓ to ½ rad per exposure. Therefore, a single fluoroscopic exam in that bygone era delivered more irradiation than the modern equipment would deliver if a woman were to have a mammogram yearly for the next twenty years. Stated another way, the total cumulative radiation exposure received by these women would be in excess of 1,000 modern mammograms.

The second report grew out of the Hiroshima-Nagasaki atom bomb disaster. Dosage of irradiation was crudely estimated depending on the distance of the exposed individuals from the center of the blast. It is estimated that the average exposure was 90 to 800 rads to the entire body. What cannot be determined with any degree of accuracy is how long these people were exposed originally or the amount of exposure to fallout in the air, in their food, their water and their surroundings. Also, the kind of irradiation produced by an atom bomb is entirely different from that which is used in modern radiological equipment. The bomb irradiation is exceedingly ''dirty'' and contains many fractions that are capable of producing mutations and cancer. Modern equipment is engineered to exclude these fractions not only in the basic machine, but also by adding sophisticated screens and filters to ensure maximum safety.

As a result of the bomb explosion, there was a measurable increase in the incidence of all types of cancer, including breast cancer. Here again, if we were to translate these crude data into an equivalent number of mammographic exposures, the range would probably be 1,600 to 2,000 mammograms. In terms of modern technology, these exposures are massive and totally unacceptable.

When we hear the word ''irradiation,'' it is extremely important to place it in its proper context. The numerals on our watches, our color television sets and the atmospheric rays emitted on a transcontinental air flight all expose us to minor amounts of irradiation. Though we use the same term, ''irradiation,'' it does not generate the same fear as when applied to the radiation from an atom bomb. We must not be carried away by our emotions or scare articles painting every aspect of this picture with the same brush without reason and without regard for the lives that may be squandered by delaying a critical diagnostic procedure.

It must be remembered that of all the asymptomatic cancers found in the breast screening program of the

Health Insurance Plan initiated by Dr. Philip Strax and supported by the National Cancer Institute, one-third were neither felt nor seen by the examiners but were discovered solely by mammography. This is truly food for thought when we must assess the life-saving benefits against the minimal risks of this most valuable diagnostic tool.

THERMOGRAPHY

In his quest for an effective, noninvasive, nonirradiation technique to diagnose breast abnormalities, the physician has utilized several other helpful diagnostic procedures. Among these is the thermogram, which is basically an infrared photograph of the breast. There is no x-ray or other ionizing irradiation involved. The thermogram simply tells us the location of any "hot spots" on the breasts. It is assumed that any new growth will generate a new blood supply and therefore will be warmer than the surrounding breast tissue. The thermogram cannot differentiate the cause for the increase in heat. A scratch on the skin, a mosquito bite, a pimple, a sunburn, an underlying pleurisy or bronchitis and even the variable times in the menstrual period are all capable of registering changes in the thermogram. It is readily clear, then, that we cannot expect a specific diagnostic answer from a nonspecific test. The thermogram is a valuable adjunct for the patient at risk when comparison tests are performed under ideal circumstances and where all possible variables have been eliminated.

Despite the fact that the thermogram is primarily a method for discovering "hot spots" in the breast, it has certain very valuable clinical applications. Not only should the thermogram findings be consistent from test to test, but they should also be symmetrical from breast to breast. Whenever an unexplainable "change" occurs, whereby a new hot spot develops asymmetrically, a warning flag should appear indicating that this finding warrants a xeromammography and/or further investigative measures.

Extensive research, particularly in Europe, has been carried out in an effort to define the various risk factors, or "predictors," of breast cancer. Those individuals in whom one or more of these risk factors are present can then be kept under closer surveillance. Many of these risk factors, such as family history of breast cancer, history of mastectomy or other reproductive system cancer (cervix, uterus or ovary), genetics, overweight, diabetes, absence of pregnancies, absence of breast-feeding, and so on, have been proposed and studied. The absolute values of many of these factors are uncertain. The questionable thermogram has been added to this list of risk factors and has been found to be a great asset in developing the profile of the person at higher risk.

In light of the fears and anxieties that have been generated relevant to x-ray mammography, the thermogram is an exceedingly valuable tool in discovering that individual who should have a mammography, regardless of her age, her history and the absence of other clinical findings. At this stage of the art, the thermogram cannot diagnose breast cancer, but it is a noninvasive, nonirradiation method to help us find those women in the higher-risk categories so that they can be more religious about their breast self-examination as well as keep their physicians on the alert. The thermogram does have an important role to play not only in breast screening, but also in surveillance. This role should grow in importance as we assemble more skills in the perfection of this technology and its interpretation.

SONOGRAPHY

The sonogram is a newer test that holds much promise for the future. This procedure, which is basically a miniature radar system, involves transmitting high-frequency sound waves into the breasts. The echo from these sound waves bounce off the intrinsic breast structures, making it possible for us to differentiate fluid-filled cysts from solid masses. The sound waves are printed on a photographic film to help us interpret the findings. Since this technique is still in its infancy, much refinement will be necessary before it will even begin to tell us what we are now able to learn from the xeromammogram.

CHAPTER 7
RECORD KEEPING

I n past generations, the covers and flyleafs of the family Bible were frequently used as the "library" for recording important events, illnesses, etc., for the entire family. This practice is commendable and certainly should be encouraged. There are many occasions when a patient must make a long-distance phone call, as far as 3,000 miles, to ask Mom when a shot was given or whether a certain childhood illness occurred. Mom might not be there to answer those questions. It is a good practice to keep a medical folder for each member of the family. Significant data pertaining to illnesses, operations, accidents, adverse reactions to medications, menstrual and obstetrical histories, important x-rays, etc., should be stored in this folder. This is a medical biography and may contain life-saving information.

Family medical biographical material can be of great value in pinpointing individuals who are at a higher risk than others for certain diseases. With this information, your physician is better able to concentrate on these high-risk factors and avoid, eliminate or stave off certain conditions. Daily discoveries by medical science help us to understand the causes for some illnesses. Avoiding known causative factors for certain illnesses by the persons at higher risk for these conditions might be life-saving to them.

Every woman should record somewhere in her personal medical history folder all significant data pertaining to her breasts. This data bank should contain not only her relevant history but also the family history of blood relatives. Facts in the family history that should be recorded include a list of all those individuals who have had any type of cancer, the relationship, the age when the condition was first discovered and the treatment. Any known causative factors, e.g., smoking and lung cancer, should be noted.

Significant personal medical history should contain the age at which menses began, a listing of any menstrual problems and data on the menopause. The use of birth-control pills, hormones and related drugs, including the dosage and duration of usage, is important. The number of pregnancies, age at the time of each pregnancy and breast-feeding history should be noted. Complications including breast abscesses, mastitis and other infections are also important. Damage to the breasts such as burns, severe impact injuries, contusions, crush injuries, lacerations, etc., should be noted, with dates where possible. Breast surgery including biopsy, "lumpectomy," excision of cysts or tumors, augmentation or reduction mammoplasties and injection of augmentation substances are all important. Where possible, record the date, physician and hospital.

X-ray can be our very best friend or our very worst enemy. It is important to record the dates and types of all x-rays, including dental x-ray, chest x-ray and all mammography. Wherever possible, record the name and address of the radiologist and where the films are kept on file. Perhaps one of the most valuable documents in this file would be a copy of a xeromammogram of the baseline condition of your breasts. If it is at all possible to acquire a duplicate of your own records, do so. If you should discover something in your breasts five years from now, reference to a baseline mammogram verifying that the identical condition was present at the time it was taken may spare you an operation plus an unnecessary nightmare.

CHAPTER 8
SUMMING UP

Important Facts for Survival in Our War Against Breast Cancer

1. Examine your breasts regularly at least once each month.

2. Have your physician perform a thorough breast examination at least once a year, preferably at the time of your gynecological exam and Pap test, and check all unusual findings without delay.

3. *Change* should be the most important word in your breast vocabulary. Have your physician evaluate even minor changes in either the appearance or the feel of your breasts.

4. If something new is found in one breast, immediately check the exact same area in the opposite breast. If the same identical finding is noted in the same areas of both breasts, it is of less significance than if it is present in only one breast. If in doubt, have it checked by your physician.

5. Eighty-percent of all lumps removed from the breast are harmless. Do not delay. The odds are in your favor.

6. The only positive way to determine the exact nature of a breast lump is through tissue biopsy and microscopic examination.

7. Do not be frightened or misled by sensationalism in the media. When in doubt, consult your physician.

8. Mammography is capable of detecting many problems that cannot be felt or seen. Let your physician be the judge of the need for this procedure.

9. Keep accurate records of significant medical data. Include dates and type of all x-rays and always know where your records are.

10. If a breast cancer is small and if it has not spread, the 10-year cure rate is approximately 90 percent. This shows the value of early detection and treatment, and underscores the importance of breast self-examination.

11. Spend as much time looking at your breasts as you do at your face. Sometimes minor clues may be *seen* before a lump can be felt. Look for changes such as dimples, indentations, retractions, bulges, distortions, change in nipple axis, recent nipple inversions, secretions and ulcerations.

12. Check your clothing for bloody discharges or secretions from the nipple.

13. Most important, consult your physician whenever in doubt. DO NOT DELAY. Breast cancer gives favor to no one.

Monthly Checklist

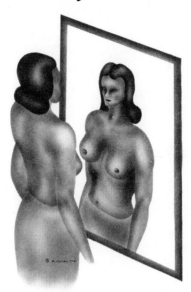

A. WHEN?

1. Once each month
   a. In the morning, when you have some privacy
   b. If menstruating, the first week after period is over
   c. If postmenopausal or post-hysterectomy, first day of the calendar month
2. Examination by doctor
   a. At least once each year
   b. If "at risk," once every six months or more often if indicated
   c. *Any time* a worrisome clue is detected

B. WHERE?

1. Privacy of your home—preferably the bedroom, where you will not be disturbed
2. Availability of large mirror—dresser or wall type
3. In the shower for first part of exam

C. HOW?

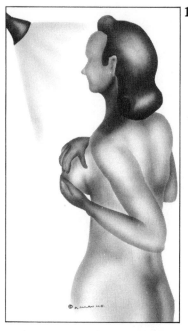

1. PALPATE BREASTS WHILE TAKING SHOWER

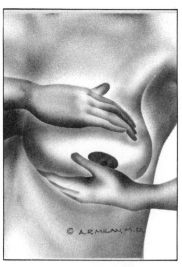

a. Use both hands if breasts are large or pendulous

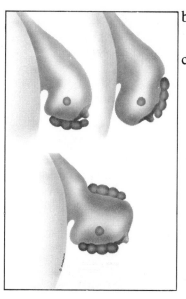

b. Press breast against chest wall

c. Use opposite hand to examine opposite breast

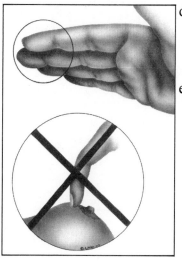

d. Feel with pads of fingers Immobilize skin with fingertips; move skin over underlying structures

e. Use two or three fingers together

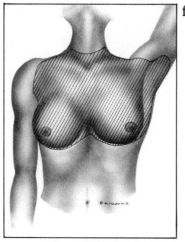

f. Examine area from neck to under portion of breast and from armpit to breastbone

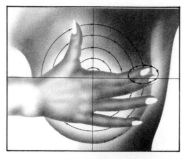

g. Examine entire breast area with concentric circle patterns

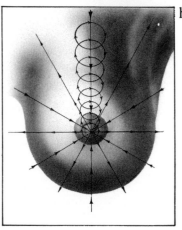

h. The twelve-stroke "clock" method may be used as an alternative

2. LIE DOWN ON BED OR COUCH

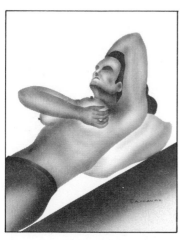

a. Place pillow or folded towels under shoulder of breast being examined

b. Place arm of side of breast being examined over forehead

c. Examine breast with pads of fingertips (two or three fingers together) of opposite hand

d. Use circular or twelve-stroke pattern

e. Place arm at side and repeat procedure

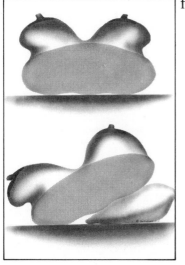

f. Place pillow under opposite shoulder, position arm similarly and examine other breast in same manner

3. OBSERVATION

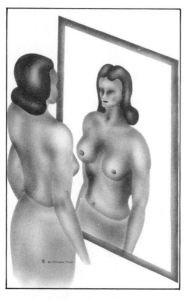

a. Stand erect before mirror, arms relaxed at sides; inspect, first looking straight ahead, then turning slowly from side to side

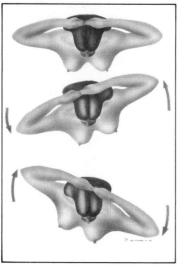

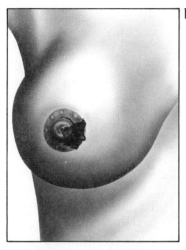

b. Inspect nipples for:

   (1) ulcers, eczema, sebaceous cyst, or other skin conditions

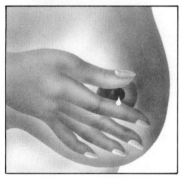

   (2) bleeding or discharge from nipples; gently try to express some secretions from nipples

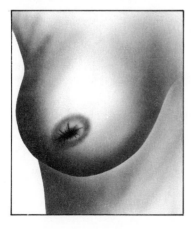

   (3) a change in shape of the nipple or areola

     (a) flattening

     (b) inversion

     (c) dimpling or retraction

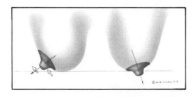

(4) a change in the nipple axis

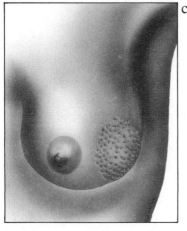

c. Examine skin surface of breast

(1) Is there any "orange peel" skin change?

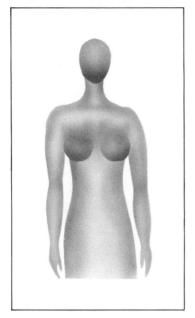

(2) Is there any change in breast contour?

(3) Is there any flattening, indentation, retraction, bulging?

(4) Is there any change in nipple axis?

(5) Does the nipple appear to be in a different position from its previous situation—i.e., is it higher, lower, pushed inward or outward?

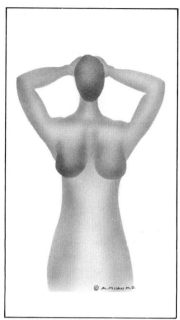

e. Raise arms above head

    (1) Place hands behind head, elbows back; inspect carefully, facing mirror directly, then while rotating each shoulder forward; look for same features as noted above

f. Pectoral contraction maneuvers

    (1) Squeeze palms together in front of forehead and hold position to tighten chest muscles on which breasts are situated; inspect carefully while facing mirror, then turn slowly from side to side

      Look for:

    (a) indentations, retractions, dimples, bulges, change in contour

    (b) change in nipple axis

    (c) distortion of breast shape not previously noted

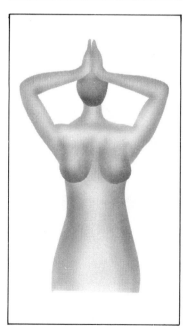

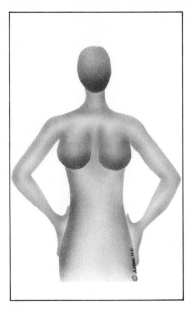

(2) Place flat of palms on hips, squeeze tightly and hold; inspect carefully while facing mirror, then while turning from side to side, observing for same features as noted above; pay particular attention to sides and under surfaces of breasts while turning from side to side

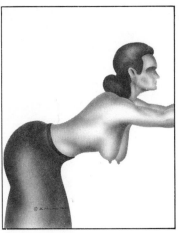

g. Leaning forward position

(1) While standing before large mirror, stretch arms forward with hands held straight out or rested on two chairs or on knees; observe carefully for a change from what has always been normal for you

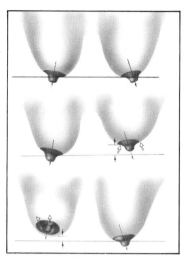

(a) are there any new dimples?

(b) are there any sores or ulcers?

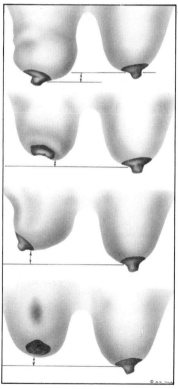

(c) is there any evidence of flattening, indentation or retraction that has not been noted previously?

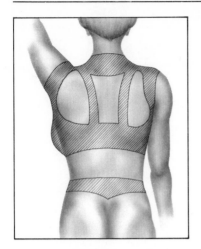

(d) are there any moles in the necklace, bra strap, sleeve or belt areas? Have they enlarged, become darker or changed in any way?

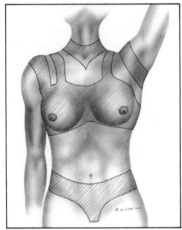

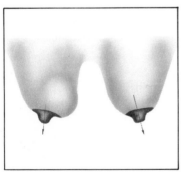

d. Shape and contour

(1) Does one breast appear to have gotten larger or smaller disproportionately?

OBSERVATIONS

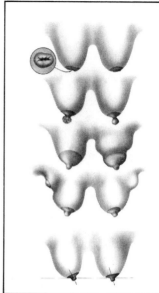

(a) Do both breasts appear to be the same size?

(b) Does a nipple invert when you lean forward?

(c) Has the nipple axis changed?

(d) Are there any new dimples, indentations, retractions, distortions or bulges?

(e) Is there any change in overall contour of either breast?

(f) Are there any new bulges in the armpit regions?

If any finding arouses doubt or suspicion, check with your doctor. To procrastinate is to invite potential disaster.